TYPE 2 DIABETES COOKBOOK

100 Recipes for Type 2 Diabetes

Table of Contents

Introduction

Type 1 diabetes (T1D) occurs when the body is unable to produce insulin, a hormone produced by the pancreas. Although the exact cause is unknown, it is believed to be a combination of genetics and environment. Today, an estimated 1.25 million people live with T1D in the United States, and 40,000 people are diagnosed every year. T1D results when the body's immune system attacks and destroys its own cells; in this case, it kills the healthy insulin-producing cells. Without insulin from these cells, the body is unable to help sugar (glucose) enter the cells to provide energy.

I wish there were another answer, but currently, management of T1D always requires insulin. Regardless of any changes you implement in your diet, vitamin intake, or lifestyle, if you are diagnosed with T1D, you will need insulin.

Insulin is an amazing hormone produced by the pancreas. The pancreas works to regulate blood sugar, or glucose, levels. It works like this: You eat something, your body digests the foods you eat, and some of that food (mostly carbohydrates but also protein and some fats) converts to glucose, which is the body's primary source of energy. Once glucose is released into the bloodstream, the pancreas responds and releases insulin, which helps move the glucose into our cells for energy. With type 1 diabetes, an outside source of insulin needs to be delivered to do the job; this is typically achieved by injecting insulin or by using an insulin pump. T1D differs from T2D in that in type 2, the body actually produces insulin, but often the insulin that is produced does not work effectively. With T2D, oral medication, non-insulin injectables, and lifestyle changes are the primary treatments

The following dietary guidelines will be helpful to anyone with type 1 diabetes.

Aim for a balanced diet. Seek out carbohydrates that are full of fiber, such as whole grains, fresh fruits, and nonprocessed vegetables. Include fish three times per week, as well as lean meats and calcium-rich protein sources, like tofu and milk. Use healthy fats, such as monounsaturated fat—these include olive and avocado oils, seeds, nuts, and nut butters. Enjoy caffeine and alcohol in moderation, limit simple sugars, and drink plenty of water.

Understand insulin action and meal timing. If you're unclear about how to time your insulin and meals, please discuss this with your diabetes educator. To be effective, insulin and meal timing need to coordinate; this will also help prevent low and high blood sugars.

Read labels. Reading labels is one of the most important things you can do in the grocery store. Become a label-reading pro! In doing so, try not to fall for any misleading claims, like those that read "sugar-free" or "no added sugar." Look at serving sizes and total grams of carbohydrates. Aim for products with at least 3 grams of fiber per 100 calories and less than 5 grams of sugar.

Include healthy proteins. Protein is essential for cell growth and repair. Include healthy, lean proteins, such as fish, tofu, or poultry. You will not take insulin to cover for protein portions unless you are eating unusually large amounts compared to your regular intake.

Carry a simple form of sugar. Keep portable snacks with you, like juice boxes, sports drinks, hard candy, jelly beans, dried fruit, honey, or glucose tablets or gels. You may need them to treat low blood sugars. Even with the best of intentions, low blood sugars can occur, so be prepared by keeping simple sugars on hand.

If you drink alcohol, eat when you do. Surprisingly, alcohol can lower blood sugars. It's always a good idea to eat some form of carbohydrates when you have a cocktail. Talk to your doctor about the best way to manage food, alcohol, and insulin.

Drink plenty of water. Is there any diet that doesn't advocate water? This diet is no different. In fact, it may be even more important for people with diabetes, since people with diabetes are at higher risk for dehydration. Don't wait until you're thirsty, and try to drink 8 to 10 glasses of water throughout the day. Also, limit beverages containing caffeine! Aim for less than 250 milligrams of caffeine daily.

Chapter 1.Breakfast

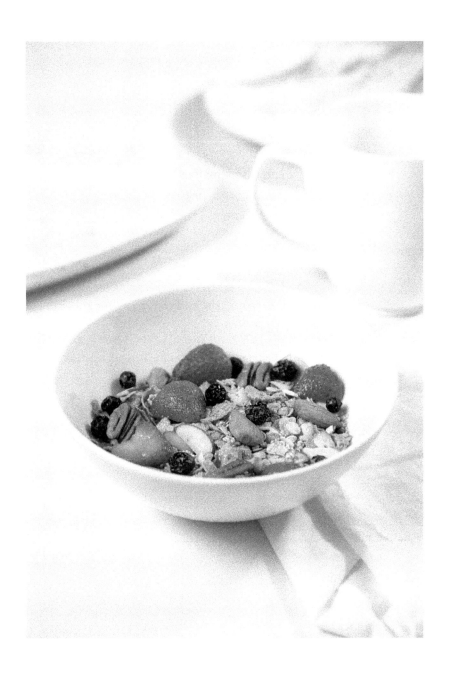

1. Cheesy Low-Carb Omelet

Preparation Time: 5 minutes
Cooking Time: 5 minutes
Servings: 5
Ingredients

- 2 whole eggs
- 1 tablespoon water
- 1 tablespoon butter
- 3 thin slices salami
- 5 fresh basil leaves
- 5 thin slices, fresh ripe tomatoes
- 2 ounces fresh mozzarella cheese
- Salt and pepper as needed

Directions:

1. Take a small bowl and whisk in eggs and water
2. Take a non-stick Sauté pan and place it over medium heat, add butter and let it melt
3. Pour egg mixture and cook for 30 seconds
4. Spread salami slices on half of egg mix and top with cheese, tomatoes, basil slices
5. Season with salt and pepper according to your taste
6. Cook for 2 minutes and fold the egg with the empty half
7. Cover and cook on LOW for 1 minute
8. Serve and enjoy!

Nutrition:

- Calories: 451
- Fat: 36g
- Carbohydrates: 3g
- Protein:33g

1. Yogurt and Kale Smoothie

Servings: 1
Preparation Time: 10 minutes
Ingredients:

- 1 cup whole milk yogurt
- 1 cup baby kale greens
- 1 pack stevia
- 1 tablespoon MCT oil
- 1 tablespoon sunflower seeds
- 1 cup of water

Directions:

1. Add listed Ingredients to the blender
2. Blend until you have a smooth and creamy texture
3. Serve chilled and enjoy!

Nutrition:

- Calories: 329
- Fat: 26g
- Carbohydrates: 15g
- Protein: 11g

2. Bacon and Chicken Garlic Wrap

Preparation Time: 15 minutes
Cooking Time: 10 minutes
Servings: 4
Ingredients

- 1 chicken fillet, cut into small cubes
- 8-9 thin slices bacon, cut to fit cubes
- 6 garlic cloves, minced

Directions:

1. Preheat your oven to 400 degrees F
2. Line a baking tray with aluminum foil
3. Add minced garlic to a bowl and rub each chicken piece with it
4. Wrap bacon piece around each garlic chicken bite

5. Secure with toothpick
6. Transfer bites to the baking sheet, keeping a little bit of space between them
7. Bake for about 15-20 minutes until crispy
8. Serve and enjoy!

Nutrition:

- Calories: 260
- Fat: 19g
- Carbohydrates: 5g
- Protein: 22g

3. Grilled Chicken Platter

Preparation Time: 5 minutes
Cooking Time: 10 minutes
Servings: 6
Ingredients

- 3 large chicken breasts, sliced half lengthwise
- 10-ounce spinach, frozen and drained
- 3-ounce mozzarella cheese, part-skim
- 1/2 a cup of roasted red peppers, cut in long strips
- 1 teaspoon of olive oil
- 2 garlic cloves, minced
- Salt and pepper as needed

Directions:

1. Preheat your oven to 400 degrees Fahrenheit
2. Slice 3 chicken breast lengthwise
3. Take a non-stick pan and grease with cooking spray
4. Bake for 2-3 minutes each side
5. Take another skillet and cook spinach and garlic in oil for 3 minutes
6. Place chicken on an oven pan and top with spinach, roasted peppers, and mozzarella
7. Bake until the cheese melted
8. Enjoy!

Nutrition:

- Calories: 195
- Fat: 7g
- Net Carbohydrates: 3g
- Protein: 30g

4. Parsley Chicken Breast

Preparation Time: 10 minutes
Cooking Time: 40 minutes
Servings: 4
Ingredients

- 1 tablespoon dry parsley
- 1 tablespoon dry basil
- 4 chicken breast halves, boneless and skinless
- 1/2 teaspoon salt
- 1/2 teaspoon red pepper flakes, crushed
- 2 tomatoes, sliced

Directions:

1. Preheat your oven to 350 degrees F
2. Take a 9x13 inch baking dish and grease it up with cooking spray
3. Sprinkle 1 tablespoon of parsley, 1 teaspoon of basil and spread the mixture over your baking dish
4. Arrange the chicken breast halves over the dish and sprinkle garlic slices on top
5. Take a small bowl and add 1 teaspoon parsley, 1 teaspoon of basil, salt, basil, red pepper and mix well. Pour the mixture over the chicken breast
6. Top with tomato slices and cover, bake for 25 minutes
7. Remove the cover and bake for 15 minutes more
8. Serve and enjoy!

Nutrition:

- Calories: 150
- Fat: 4g
- Carbohydrates: 4g
- Protein: 25g

5. Mustard Chicken

Preparation Time: 10 minutes
Cooking Time: 40 minutes
Servings: 4
Ingredients

- 4 chicken breasts
- 1/2 cup chicken broth
- 3-4 tablespoons mustard
- 3 tablespoons olive oil
- 1 teaspoon paprika
- 1 teaspoon chili powder
- 1 teaspoon garlic powder

Directions:

1. Take a small bowl and mix mustard, olive oil, paprika, chicken broth, garlic powder, chicken broth, and chili
2. Add chicken breast and marinate for 30 minutes
3. Take a lined baking sheet and arrange the chicken
4. Bake for 35 minutes at 375 degrees Fahrenheit
5. Serve and enjoy!

Nutrition:

- Calories: 531
- Fat: 23g
- Carbohydrates: 10g
- Protein: 64g

6. Balsamic Chicken

Preparation Time: 10 minutes
Cooking Time: 25 minutes
Servings: 6
Ingredients

- 6 chicken breast halves, skinless and boneless
- 1 teaspoon garlic salt
- Ground black pepper
- 2 tablespoons olive oil
- 1 onion, thinly sliced
- 14- and 1/2-ounces tomatoes, diced
- 1/2 cup balsamic vinegar
- 1 teaspoon dried basil
- 1 teaspoon dried oregano
- 1 teaspoon dried rosemary
- 1/2 teaspoon dried thyme

Directions:

1. Season both sides of your chicken breasts thoroughly with pepper and garlic salt
2. Take a skillet and place it over medium heat
3. Add some oil and cook your seasoned chicken for 3-4 minutes per side until the breasts are nicely browned
4. Add some onion and cook for another 3-4 minutes until the onions are browned
5. Pour the diced-up tomatoes and balsamic vinegar over your chicken and season with some rosemary, basil, thyme, and rosemary
6. Simmer the chicken for about 15 minutes until they are no longer pink
7. Take an instant-read thermometer and check if the internal temperature gives a reading of 165 degrees Fahrenheit
8. If yes, then you are good to go!

Nutrition:

- Calories: 196
- Fat: 7g
- Carbohydrates: 7g
- Protein: 23g

7. Greek Chicken Breast

Preparation Time: 10 minutes
Cooking Time: 25 minutes
Servings: 4
Ingredients

- 4 chicken breast halves, skinless and boneless
- 1 cup extra virgin olive oil
- 1 lemon, juiced
- 2 teaspoons garlic, crushed
- 1 and 1/2 teaspoons black pepper
- 1/3 teaspoon paprika

Directions:

1. Cut 3 slits in the chicken breast
2. Take a small bowl and whisk in olive oil, salt, lemon juice, garlic, paprika, pepper and whisk for 30 seconds
3. Place chicken in a large bowl and pour marinade
4. Rub the marinade all over using your hand
5. Refrigerate overnight
6. Pre-heat grill to medium heat and oil the grate
7. Cook chicken in the grill until center is no longer pink
8. Serve and enjoy!

Nutrition:

- Calories: 644
- Fat: 57g
- Carbohydrates: 2g
- Protein: 27g

8. Breakfast Smoothie Bowl with Fresh Berries

Preparation Time: 10 minutes
Cooking Time: 5 minutes
Servings: 2
Ingredients:

- Almond milk (unsweetened) – 1/2 cup
- Psyllium husk powder – 1/2 teaspoon
- Strawberries (chopped) – 2 ounces
- Coconut oil – 1 tablespoon
- Crushed ice – 3 cups
- Liquid stevia – 5 to 10 drops
- Pea protein powder – 1/3 cup

Directions:

1. Begin by taking a blender and adding in the mashed ice cubes. Allow them to rest for about 30 seconds.
2. Then put in the almond milk, shredded strawberries, pea protein powder, psyllium husk powder, coconut oil, and liquid stevia. Blend well until it turns into a smooth and creamy puree.
3. Vacant the prepared smoothie into 2 glasses.
4. Cover with coconut flakes and pure and neat strawberries.

Nutrition:

- Calories: 166 calories per serving
- Fat – 9.2 g
- Carbohydrates – 4.1 g
- Protein – 17.6 g

9. Chia and Coconut Pudding

Preparation Time: 10 minutes
Cooking Time: 5 minutes
Servings: 2
Ingredients:

- Light coconut milk – 7 ounces
- Liquid stevia – 3 to 4 drops
- Kiwi – 1

17

- Chia seeds – ¼ cup
- Clementine – 1
- Shredded coconut (unsweetened)

Directions:

1. Begin by getting a mixing bowl and putting in the light coconut milk. Set in the liquid stevia to sweeten the milk. Combine well.
2. Put the chia seeds to the milk and whisk until well-combined. Arrange aside.
3. Scrape the clementine and carefully extract the skin from the wedges. Leave aside.
4. Also, scrape the kiwi and dice it into small pieces.
5. Get a glass vessel and gather the pudding. For this, position the fruits at the bottom of the jar; then put a dollop of chia pudding. Then spray the fruits and then put another layer of chia pudding.
6. Finalize by garnishing with the rest of the fruits and chopped coconut.

Nutrition:

- Calories: 201 calories per serving
- Protein – 5.4 g
- Fat – 10 g
- Carbohydrates – 22.8 g

10. Tomato and Zucchini Sauté

Preparation Time: 10 minutes
Cooking Time: 43 minutes
Servings: 6
Ingredients:

- Vegetable oil – 1 tablespoon
- Tomatoes (chopped) – 2
- Green bell pepper (chopped) – 1
- Black pepper (freshly ground) – as per taste
- Onion (sliced) – 1
- Zucchini (peeled) – 2 pounds and cut into 1-inch-thick slices

- Salt – as per taste
- Uncooked white rice – ¼ cup

Directions:
1. Begin by getting a nonstick pan and putting it over low heat. Stream in the oil and allow it to heat through.
Put in the onions and sauté for about 3 minutes.
2. Then pour in the zucchini and green peppers. Mix well and spice with black pepper and salt.
3. Reduce the heat and cover the pan with a lid. Allow the veggies cook on low for 5 minutes.
4. While you're done, put in the water and rice. Place the lid back on and cook on low for 20 minutes.

Nutrition:

- Calories: 94 calories per serving
- Fat – 2.8 g
- Protein – 3.2 g
- Carbohydrates – 16.1 g

11. Steamed Kale with Mediterranean Dressing

Preparation Time: 10 minutes
Cooking Time: 25 minutes
Servings: 6
Ingredients:
- Kale (chopped) – 12 cups
- Olive oil – 1 tablespoon
- Soy sauce – 1 teaspoon
- Pepper (freshly ground) – as per taste
- Lemon juice – 2 tablespoons
- Garlic (minced) – 1 tablespoon
- Salt – as per taste

Directions:

1. Get a gas steamer or an electric steamer and fill the bottom pan with water. If making use of a gas steamer, position it on high heat. Making use of an electric steamer, place it on the highest setting.
2. Immediately the water comes to a boil, put in the shredded kale and cover with a lid. Boil for about 8 minutes. The kale should be tender by now.
3. During the kale is boiling, take a big mixing bowl and put in the olive oil, lemon juice, soy sauce, garlic, pepper, and salt. Whisk well to mix.
4. Now toss in the steamed kale and carefully enclose into the dressing. Be assured the kale is well-coated.
5. Serve while it's hot!

Nutrition:

- Calories: 91 calories per serving
- Fat – 3.5 g
- Protein – 4.6 g
- Carbohydrates – 14.5 g

12. Healthy Carrot Muffins

Preparation Time: 10 minutes
Cooking Time: 40 minutes
Servings: 8
Ingredients:
Dry ingredients

- Tapioca starch – ¼ cup
- Baking soda – 1 teaspoon
- Cinnamon – 1 tablespoon
- Cloves – ¼ teaspoon
- Wet ingredients
- Vanilla extract – 1 teaspoon
- Water – 11/2 cups
- Carrots (shredded) – 11/2 cups
- Almond flour – 1¾ cups
- Granulated sweetener of choice – 1/2 cup
- Baking powder – 1 teaspoon

- Nutmeg – 1 teaspoon
- Salt – 1 teaspoon
- Coconut oil – 1/3 cup
- Flax meal – 4 tablespoons
- Banana (mashed) – 1 medium

Directions:

1. Begin by heating the oven to 350F.
2. Get a muffin tray and position paper cups in all the molds. Arrange aside.
3. Get a small glass bowl and put half a cup of water and flax meal. Allow this rest for about 5 minutes. Your flax egg is prepared.
4. Get a large mixing bowl and put in the almond flour, tapioca starch, granulated sugar, baking soda, baking powder, cinnamon, nutmeg, cloves, and salt. Mix well to combine.
5. Conform a well in the middle of the flour mixture and stream in the coconut oil, vanilla extract, and flax egg. Mix well to conform a mushy dough. Then put in the chopped carrots and mashed banana. Mix until well-combined.
6. Make use of a spoon to scoop out an equal amount of mixture into 8 muffin cups.
7. Position the muffin tray in the oven and allow it to bake for about 40 minutes.
8. Extract the tray from the microwave and allow the muffins to stand for about 10 minutes.
9. Extract the muffin cups from the tray and allow them to chill until they reach room degree of hotness and coldness.
10. Serve and enjoy!

Nutrition:

- Calories: 189 calories per serving
- Fat – 13.9 g
- Protein – 3.8 g
- Carbohydrates – 17.3 g

13. Vegetable Noodles Stir-Fry

Preparation Time: 10 minutes
Cooking Time: 40 minutes
Servings: 4
Ingredients:

- White sweet potato – 1 pound
- Zucchini – 8 ounces
- Garlic cloves (finely chopped) – 2 larges
- Vegetable broth – 2 tablespoons
- Salt – as per taste
- Carrots – 8 ounces
- Shallot (finely chopped) – 1
- Red chili (finely chopped) – 1
- Olive oil – 1 tablespoon
- Pepper – as per taste

Directions:

1. Begin by scrapping the carrots and sweet potato. Make Use a spiralizer to make noodles out of the sweet potato and carrots.
2. Rinse the zucchini thoroughly and spiralize it as well.
3. Get a large skillet and position it on a high flame. Stream in the vegetable broth and allow it to come to a boil.
4. Toss in the spiralized sweet potato and carrots. Then put in the chili, garlic, and shallots. Stir everything using tongs and cook for some minutes.
5. Transfer the vegetable noodles into a serving platter and generously spice with pepper and salt.
6. Finalize by sprinkling olive oil over the noodles. Serve while hot!

Nutrition:

- Calories: 169 calories per serving
- Fat – 3.7 g
- Protein – 3.6 g
- Carbohydrates – 31.2 g

14. Berry-Oat Breakfast Bars

Preparation Time: 10 minutes
Cooking Time: 25 minutes
Servings: 12
Ingredients:

- 2 cups fresh raspberries or blueberries
- 2 tablespoons sugar
- 2 tablespoons freshly squeezed lemon juice
- 1 tablespoon cornstarch
- 1 1/2 cups rolled oats
- 1/2 cup whole-wheat flour
- 1/2 cup walnuts
- ¼ cup chia seeds
- ¼ cup extra-virgin olive oil
- ¼ cup honey
- 1 large egg

Directions:

1. Preheat the oven to 350f.
2. In a small saucepan over medium heat, stir together the berries, sugar, lemon juice, and cornstarch. Bring to a simmer. Reduce the heat and simmer for 2 to 3 minutes, until the mixture thickens.
3. In a food processor or high-speed blender, combine the oats, flour, walnuts, and chia seeds. Process until powdered. Add the olive oil, honey, and egg. Pulse a few more times, until well combined. Press half of the mixture into a 9-inch square baking dish.
4. Spread the berry filling over the oat mixture. Add the remaining oat mixture on top of the berries. Bake for 25 minutes, until browned.
5. Let cool completely, cut into 12 pieces, and serve. Store in a covered container for up to 5 days.

Nutrition:

- calories: 201; total fat: 10g; saturated fat: 1g; protein: 5g; carbs: 26g; sugar: 9g; fiber: 5g; cholesterol: 16mg; sodium: 8mg

30 minutes or less • nut free • vegetarian

15. Whole-Grain Breakfast Cookies

Preparation Time: 20 minutes
Cooking Time: 10 minutes
Servings: 18 cookies
Ingredients:

- 2 cups rolled oats
- 1/2 cup whole-wheat flour
- ¼ cup ground flaxseed
- 1 teaspoon baking powder
- 1 cup unsweetened applesauce
- 2 large eggs
- 2 tablespoons vegetable oil
- 2 teaspoons vanilla extract
- 1 teaspoon ground cinnamon
- 1/2 cup dried cherries
- ¼ cup unsweetened shredded coconut
- 2 ounces dark chocolate, chopped

Directions:

1. Preheat the oven to 350f.
2. In a large bowl, combine the oats, flour, flaxseed, and baking powder. Stir well to mix.
3. In a medium bowl, whisk the applesauce, eggs, vegetable oil, vanilla, and cinnamon. Pour the wet mixture into the dry mix, and stir until just combined.
4. Fold in the cherries, coconut, and chocolate. Drop tablespoon-size balls of dough onto a baking sheet. Bake for 10 to 12 minutes, until browned and cooked through.
5. Let cool for about 3 minutes, remove from the baking sheet, and cool completely before serving. Store in an airtight container for up to 1 week.

Nutrition:

- Calories: 136;
- Total fat: 7g;
- Saturated fat: 3g;
- Protein: 4g;
- Carbs: 14g;
- Sugar: 4g;
- Fiber: 3g;
- Cholesterol: 21mg;
- Sodium: 11mg

Chapter 2.Lunch

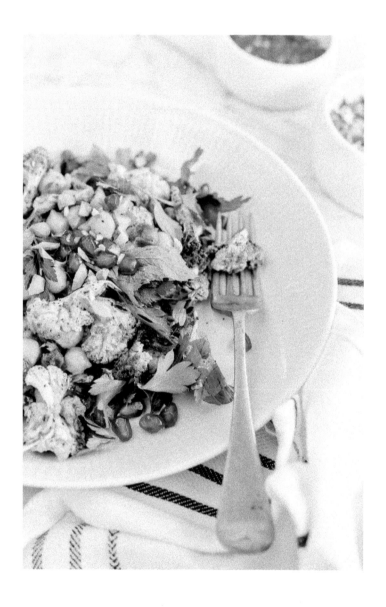

16. Chicken, Strawberry, And Avocado Salad

Preparation Time: 10 Minutes
Cooking Time: 5 Minutes
Ingredients

- 1,5 cups chicken (skin removed)
- 1/4 cup almonds
- 2 (5-oz) pkg salad greens
- 1 (16-oz) pkg strawberries
- 1 avocado
- 1/4 cup green onion
- 1/4 cup lime juice
- 3 tbsp. extra virgin olive oil
- 2 tbsp. honey
- 1/4 tsp. salt
- 1/4 tsp. pepper

Directions

1. Toast almonds until golden and fragrant.
2. Mix lime juice, oil, honey, salt, and pepper.
3. Mix greens, sliced strawberries, chicken, diced avocado, and sliced green onion and sliced almonds; drizzle with dressing. Toss to coat.

Nutrition:

- Calories 150
- Protein 15 g
- Fat 10 g, Carbs 5 g

17. Lemon-Thyme Eggs

Preparation Time: 10 Minutes
Cooking Time: 5 Minutes
Servings: 4

Ingredients

- 7 large eggs
- 1/4 cup mayonnaise (reduced-fat)
- 2 tsp. lemon juice
- 1 tsp. Dijon mustard
- 1 tsp. chopped fresh thyme
- 1/8 tsp. cayenne pepper

Directions

1. Bring eggs to a boil.
2. Peel and cut each egg in half lengthwise.
3. Remove yolks to a bowl. Add mayonnaise, lemon juice, mustard, thyme, and cayenne to egg yolks; mash to blend. Fill egg white halves with yolk mixture.
4. Chill until ready to serve.

Nutrition:

- Calories 40
- Protein 10 g
- Fat 6 g
- Carbs 2 g

18. Spinach Salad with Bacon

Preparation Time: 15 Minutes
Cooking Time: 0 Minutes
Servings: 4

Ingredients:

- 8 slices center-cut bacon
- 3 tbsp. extra virgin olive oil
- 1 (5-oz) pkg baby spinach
- 1 tbsp. apple cider vinegar
- 1 tsp. Dijon mustard
- 1/2 tsp. honey
- 1/4 tsp. salt
- 1/2 tsp. pepper

Directions:

1. Mix vinegar, mustard, honey, salt and pepper in a bowl.
2. Whisk in oil. Place spinach in a serving bowl; drizzle with dressing, and toss to coat.
3. Sprinkle with cooked and crumbled bacon.

Nutrition:

- Calories 110
- Protein 6 g
- Fat 2 g
- Carbs 1 g

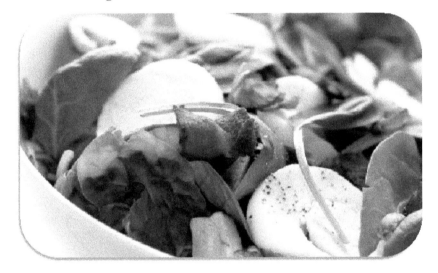

19. Pea and Collards Soup

Preparation Time: 10 Minutes
Cooking Time: 50 Minutes
Servings: 4
Ingredients

- 1/2 (16-oz) pkg black-eyed peas
- 1 onion
- 2 carrots
- 1,5 cups ham (low-sodium)
- 1 (1-lb) bunch collard greens (trimmed)
- 1 tbsp. extra virgin olive oil
- 2 cloves garlic

- 1/2 tsp. black pepper
- Hot sauce

Directions
1. Cook chopped onion and carrots 10 Minutes.
2. Add peas, diced ham, collards, and Minced garlic. Cook 5 Minutes.
3. Add broth, 3 cups water, and pepper. Bring to a boil; simmer 35 Minutes, adding water if needed.
4. Serve with favorite sauce.

Nutrition:

- Calories 86
- Protein 15 g
- Fat 2 g
- Carbs 9 g

20. Spanish Stew
Preparation Time: 10 Minutes
Cooking Time: 25 Minutes
Servings: 4
Ingredients
- 1.1/2 (12-oz) pkg smoked chicken sausage links
- 1 (5-oz) pkg baby spinach
- 1 (15-oz) can chickpeas
- 1 (14.5-oz) can tomatoes with basil, garlic, and oregano
- 1/2 tsp. smoked paprika
- 1/2 tsp. cumin
- 3/4 cup onions
- 1 tbsp. extra virgin olive oil

Directions
1. Cook sliced the sausage in hot oil until browned. Remove from pot.
2. Add chopped onions; cook until tender.

3. Add sausage, drained and rinsed chickpeas, diced tomatoes, paprika, and ground cumin. Cook 15 Minutes.
4. Add in spinach; cook 1 to 2 Minutes.

Nutrition:

- Calories 200
- Protein 10 g
- Fat 20 g
- Carbs 1 g

21. Creamy Taco Soup

Preparation Time: 10 Minutes
Cooking Time: 20 Minutes
Servings: 4
Ingredients

- 3/4 lb. ground sirloin
- 1/2 (8-oz) cream cheese
- 1/2 onion
- 1 clove garlic
- 1 (10-oz) can tomatoes and green chiles
- 1 (14.5-oz) can beef broth
- 1/4 cup heavy cream
- 1,5 tsp. cumin
- 1/2 tsp. chili powder

Directions

1. Cook beef, chopped onion, and Minced garlic until meat is browned and crumbly; drain and return to pot.
2. Add ground cumin, chili powder, and cream cheese cut into small pieces and softened, stirring until cheese is melted.
3. Add diced tomatoes, broth, and cream; bring to a boil, and simmer 10 Minutes. Season with pepper and salt to taste.

Nutrition:

- Calories 60

- Protein 3 g
- Fat 1 g
- Carbs 8 g

22. Chicken with Caprese Salsa

Preparation Time: 15 Minutes
Cooking Time: 5 Minutes
Servings: 4
Ingredients

- 3/4 lb. boneless, skinless chicken breasts
- 2 big tomatoes
- 1/2 (8-oz) ball fresh mozzarella cheese
- 1/4 cup red onion
- 2 tbsp. fresh basil
- 1 tbsp. balsamic vinegar
- 2 tbsp. extra virgin olive oil (divided)
- 1/2 tsp. salt (divided)
- 1/4 tsp. pepper (divided)

Directions

1. Sprinkle cut in half lengthwise chicken with 1/4 tsp. salt and 1/8 tsp. pepper.
2. Heat 1 tbsp. olive oil, cook chicken 5 Minutes.
3. Meanwhile, mix chopped tomatoes, diced cheese, finely chopped onion, chopped basil, vinegar, 1 tbsp. oil, and 1/4 tsp. salt and 1/8 tsp. pepper.
4. Spoon salsa over chicken.

Nutrition:

- Calories 210
- Protein 28 g
- Fat 17 g
- Carbs 0, 1 g

23. Balsamic-Roasted Broccoli

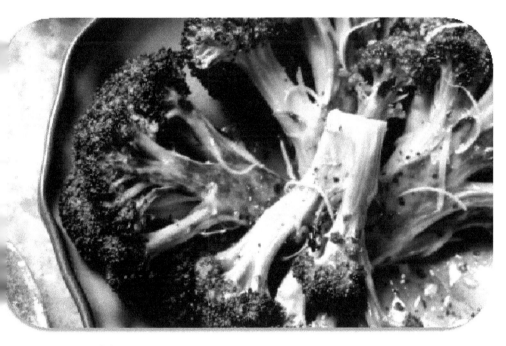

Preparation Time: 10 Minutes
Cooking Time: 15 Minutes
Servings: 4
Ingredients

- 1 lb. broccoli
- 1 tbsp. extra virgin olive oil
- 1 tbsp. balsamic vinegar
- 1 clove garlic
- 1/8 tsp. salt
- Pepper to taste

Directions
1. Preheat oven to 450F.

2. Combine broccoli, olive oil, vinegar, Minced garlic, salt, and pepper; toss.
3. Spread broccoli on a baking sheet.
4. Bake 12 to 15 Minutes.

Nutrition:

- Calories 27
- Protein 3 g
- Fat 0, 3 g
- Carbs 4 g

24. Hearty Beef and Vegetable Soup

Preparation Time: 10 Minutes
Cooking Time: 30 Minutes
Servings: 4
Ingredients

- 1/2 lb. lean ground beef
- 2 cups beef broth
- 1,5 tbsp. vegetable oil (divided)
- 1 cup green bell pepper
- 1/2 cup red onion
- 1 cup green cabbage
- 1 cup frozen mixed vegetables
- 1/2 can tomatoes
- 1,5 tsp. Worcestershire sauce
- 1 small bay leaf
- 1,8 tsp. pepper
- 2 tbsp. ketchup

Directions

1. Cook beef in 1/2 tbsp. hot oil 2 Minutes.
2. Stir in chopped bell pepper and chopped onion; cook 4 Minutes.
3. Add chopped cabbage, mixed vegetables, stewed tomatoes, broth, Worcestershire sauce, bay leaf, and pepper; bring to a boil.
4. Reduce heat to medium; cover, and cook 15 Minutes.

5. Stir in ketchup and 1 tbsp. oil, and remove from heat. Let stand 10 Minutes.

Nutrition:

- Calories 170
- Protein 17 g
- Fat 8 g
- Carbs 3 g

25. Cauliflower Muffin

Preparation Time: 15 Minutes
Cooking Time: 30 Minutes
Servings: 4
Ingredients

- 2,5 cup cauliflower
- 2/3 cup ham
- 2,5 cups of cheese
- 2/3 cup champignon
- 1,5 tbsp. flaxseed
- 3 eggs
- 1/4 tsp. salt
- 1/8 tsp. pepper

Directions

1. 1. Preheat oven to 375 F.
2. Put muffin liners in a 12-muffin tin.
3. Combine diced cauliflower, ground flaxseed, beaten eggs, cup diced ham, grated cheese, and diced mushrooms, salt, pepper.
4. Divide mixture rightly between muffin liners.
5. Bake 30 Minutes.

Nutrition:

- Calories 116
- Protein 10 g

- Fat 7 g
- Carbs 3 g

26. Ham and Egg Cups

Preparation Time: 10 Minutes
Cooking Time: 15 Minutes
Servings: 4
Ingredients

- 5 slices ham
- 4 tbsp. cheese
- 1,5 tbsp. cream
- 3 egg whites
- 1,5 tbsp. pepper (green)
- 1 tsp. salt
- pepper to taste

Directions

1. Preheat oven to 350 F.
2. Arrange each slice of thinly sliced ham into 4 muffin tin.
3. Put 1/4 of grated cheese into ham cup.
4. Mix eggs, cream, salt and pepper and divide it into 2 tins.
5. Bake in oven 15 Minutes; after baking, sprinkle with green onions.

Nutrition:

- Calories 180
- Protein 13 g
- Fat 13 g
- Carbs 2 g

27. Cauliflower Rice with Chicken

Preparation Time: 15 Minutes
Cooking Time: 15 Minutes
Servings: 4

Ingredients

- 1/2 large cauliflower
- 3/4 cup cooked meat
- 1/2 bell pepper
- 1 carrot
- 2 ribs celery
- 1 tbsp. stir fry sauce (low carb)
- 1 tbsp. extra virgin olive oil
- Salt and pepper to taste

Directions

1. Chop cauliflower in a processor to "rice." Place in a bowl.
2. Properly chop all vegetables in a food processor into thin slices.
3. Add cauliflower and other plants to WOK with heated oil. Fry until all veggies are tender.
4. Add chopped meat and sauce to the wok and fry 10 Minutes.
5. Serve.

Nutrition:

- Calories 200
- Protein 10 g
- Fat 12 g
- Carbs 10 g

28. Turkey with Fried Eggs

Preparation Time: 10 Minutes
Cooking Time: 20 Minutes
Servings: 4
Ingredients

- 4 large potatoes
- 1 cooked turkey thigh
- 1 large onion (about 2 cups diced)
- butter
- Chile flakes
- 4 eggs

- salt to taste
- pepper to taste

Directions
1. Rub the cold boiled potatoes on the coarsest holes of a box grater. Dice the turkey.
2. Cook the onion in as much unsalted butter as you feel comfortable with until it's just fragrant and translucent.
3. Add the rubbed potatoes and a cup of diced cooked turkey, salt and pepper to taste, and cook 20 Minutes.

Nutrition:

- Calories 170
- Protein 19 g
- Fat 7 g
- Carbs 6 g

29. Shredded Chicken Salad

Preparation Time: 5 minutes
Cooking Time: 10 minutes
Servings: 6
Ingredients:

- 2 chicken breasts, boneless, skinless
- 1 head iceberg lettuce, cut into strips
- 2 bell peppers, cut into strips
- 1 fresh cucumber, quartered, sliced
- 3 scallions, sliced
- 2 tbsp. chopped peanuts
- 1 tbsp. peanut vinaigrette
- Salt to taste
- 1 cup water

Directions:
1. In a skillet simmer one cup of salted water.

2. Add the chicken breasts, cover and cook on low for 5 minutes. Remove the cover. Then remove the chicken from the skillet and shred with a fork.
3. In a salad bowl mix the vegetables with the cooled chicken, season with salt and sprinkle with peanut vinaigrette and chopped peanuts.

Nutrition:

- Carbohydrates: 9 g
- Protein: 11.6 g
- Total sugars: 4.2 g
- Calories: 117

30. Broccoli Salad

Preparation Time: 10 minutes
Cooking Time: none
Servings: 6
Ingredients:

- 1 medium head broccoli, raw, florets only
- 1/2 cup red onion, chopped
- 12 oz. turkey bacon, chopped, fried until crisp
- 1/2 cup cherry tomatoes, halved
- ¼ cup sunflower kernels
- ¾ cup raisins
- ¾ cup mayonnaise
- 2 tbsp. white vinegar

Directions:

1. In a salad bowl combine the broccoli, tomatoes and onion.
2. Mix mayo with vinegar and sprinkle over the broccoli.
3. Add the sunflower kernels, raisins and bacon and toss well.

Nutrition:

- Carbohydrates: 17.3 g
- Protein: 11 g
- Total sugars: 10 g

- Calories: 220

31. Cherry Tomato Salad

Preparation Time: 10 minutes
Cooking Time: none
Servings: 6
Ingredients:

- 40 cherry tomatoes, halved
- 1 cup mozzarella balls, halved
- 1 cup green olives, sliced
- 1 can (6 oz.) black olives, sliced
- 2 green onions, chopped
- 3 oz. roasted pine nuts
- Dressing:
- 1/2 cup olive oil
- 2 tbsp. red wine vinegar
- 1 tsp. dried oregano
- Salt and pepper to taste

Directions:
1. In a salad bowl, combine the tomatoes, olives and onions.
2. Prepare the dressing by combining olive oil with red wine vinegar, dried oregano, salt and pepper.
3. Sprinkle with the dressing and add the nuts.
4. Let marinate in the fridge for 1 hour.

Nutrition:

- Carbohydrates: 10.7 g, Protein: 2.4 g, Total sugars: 3.6 g

32. Sweet Potato, Kale, and White Bean Stew

Preparation Time: 15 minutes
Cooking Time: 25 minutes
Servings: 4

Ingredients:
- 1 (15-ounce) can low-sodium cannellini beans, rinsed and drained, divided
- 1 tablespoon olive oil
- 1 medium onion, chopped
- 2 garlic cloves, minced
- 2 celery stalks, chopped
- 3 medium carrots, chopped
- 2 cups low-sodium vegetable broth
- 1 teaspoon apple cider vinegar
- 2 medium sweet potatoes (about 1¼ pounds)
- 2 cups chopped kale
- 1 cup shelled edamame
- ¼ cup quinoa
- 1 teaspoon dried thyme
- 1/2 teaspoon cayenne pepper
- 1/2 teaspoon salt
- ¼ teaspoon freshly ground black pepper

Directions:
1. Put half the beans into a blender and blend until smooth. Set aside.
2. In a large soup pot over medium heat, heat the oil. When the oil is shining, include the onion and garlic, and cook until the onion softens. The garlic is sweet, about 3 minutes. Add the celery and carrots, and continue cooking until the vegetables soften, about 5 minutes.
3. Add the broth, vinegar, sweet potatoes, unblended beans, kale, edamame, and quinoa, and bring the mixture to a boil. Reduce the heat and simmer until the vegetables soften, about 10 minutes.
4. Add the blended beans, thyme, cayenne, salt, and black pepper, increase the heat to medium-high, and bring the mixture to a boil. Reduce the heat and simmer, uncovered, until the flavors combine, about 5 minutes.
5. Into each of 4 containers, scoop 1¾ cups of stew.

Nutrition:

- calories: 373; total fat: 7g
- saturated fat: 1g; protein: 15g
- total carbs: 65g; fiber: 15g
- sugar: 13g; sodium: 540mg

33. Slow Cooker Two-Bean Sloppy Joes

Preparation Time: 10 minutes
Cooking Time: 6 hours
Servings: 4
Ingredients:

- 1 (15-ounce) can low-sodium black beans
- 1 (15-ounce) can low-sodium pinto beans
- 1 (15-ounce) can no-salt-added diced tomatoes
- 1 medium green bell pepper, cored, seeded, and chopped
- 1 medium yellow onion, chopped
- ¼ cup low-sodium vegetable broth
- 2 garlic cloves, minced
- 2 servings (¼ cup) meal prep barbecue sauce or bottled barbecue sauce
- ¼ teaspoon salt
- ¼ teaspoon freshly ground black pepper
- 4 whole-wheat buns

Directions:

1. In a slow cooker, combine the black beans, pinto beans, diced tomatoes, bell pepper, onion, broth, garlic, meal prep barbecue sauce, salt, and black pepper. Stir the ingredients, then cover and cook on low for 6 hours.
2. Into each of 4 containers, spoon 1¼ cups of sloppy joe mix. Serve with 1 whole-wheat bun.
3. Storage: place airtight containers in the refrigerator for up to 1 week. To freeze, place freezer-safe containers in the freezer for up to 2 months. To defrost, refrigerate overnight. To reheat individual portions, microwave uncovered on high for 2 to 21/2 minutes. Alternatively, reheat the entire dish in a saucepan on the stove top. Bring the sloppy joes to a boil, then reduce the heat

and simmer until heated through, 10 to 15 minutes. Serve with a whole-wheat bun.

Nutrition:

- calories: 392; total fat: 3g
- saturated fat: 0g; protein: 17g
- total carbs: 79g; fiber: 19g
- sugar: 15g; sodium: 759mg

34. Lighter Eggplant Parmesan

Preparation Time: 15 minutes
Cooking Time: 35 minutes
Servings: 4
Ingredients:
- Nonstick cooking spray
- 3 eggs, beaten
- 1 tablespoon dried parsley
- 2 teaspoons ground oregano
- 1/8 teaspoon freshly ground black pepper
- 1 cup panko bread crumbs, preferably whole-wheat
- 1 large eggplant (about 2 pounds)
- 5 servings (21/2 cups) chunky tomato sauce or jarred low-sodium tomato sauce
- 1 cup part-skim mozzarella cheese
- ¼ cup grated parmesan cheese

Directions:
1. Preheat the oven to 450f. Coat a baking sheet with cooking spray.
2. In a medium bowl, whisk together the eggs, parsley, oregano, and pepper.
3. Pour the panko into a separate medium bowl.
4. Slice the eggplant into ¼-inch-thick slices. Dip each slice of eggplant into the egg mixture, shaking off the excess. Then

dredge both sides of the eggplant in the panko bread crumbs. Place the coated eggplant on the prepared baking sheet, leaving a 1/2-inch space between each slice.

5. Bake for about 15 minutes until soft and golden brown. Remove from the oven and set aside to slightly cool.

6. Pour 1/2 cup of chunky tomato sauce on the bottom of an 8-by-15-inch baking dish. Using a spatula or the back of a spoon spread the tomato sauce evenly. Place half the slices of cooked eggplant, slightly overlapping, in the dish, and top with 1 cup of chunky tomato sauce, 1/2 cup of mozzarella and 2 tablespoons of grated parmesan. Repeat the layer, ending with the cheese.

7. Bake uncovered for 20 minutes until the cheese is bubbling and slightly browned.

8. Remove from the oven and allow cooling for 15 minutes before dividing the eggplant equally into 4 separate containers.

Nutrition:

- calories: 333; total fat: 14g
- saturated fat: 6g; protein: 20g
- total carbs: 35g; fiber: 11g
- sugar: 15g; sodium: 994mg

35. Coconut-Lentil Curry

Preparation Time: 15 minutes
Cooking Time: 35 minutes
Servings: 4
Ingredients:

- 1 tablespoon olive oil
- 1 medium yellow onion, chopped
- 1 garlic clove, minced
- 1 medium red bell pepper, diced
- 1 (15-ounce) can green or brown lentils, rinsed and drained
- 2 medium sweet potatoes, washed, peeled, and cut into bite-size chunks (about 1¼ pounds)
- 1 (15-ounce) can no-salt-added diced tomatoes
- 2 tablespoons tomato paste
- 4 teaspoons curry powder

- 1/8 teaspoon ground cloves
- 1 (15-ounce) can light coconut milk
- ¼ teaspoon salt
- 2 pieces whole-wheat naan bread, halved, or 4 slices crusty bread

Directions:
1. In a large saucepan over medium heat, heat the olive oil. When the oil is shimmering, add both the onion and garlic and cook until the onion softens. The garlic is sweet, for about 3 minutes.
2. Add the bell pepper and continue cooking until it softens, about 5 minutes more. Add the lentils, sweet potatoes, tomatoes, tomato paste, curry powder, and cloves, and bring the mixture to a boil. Reduce the heat to medium-low, cover, and simmer until the potatoes are softened, about 20 minutes.
3. Add the coconut milk and salt, and return to a boil. Reduce the heat and simmer until the flavors combine, about 5 minutes.
4. Into each of 4 containers, spoon 2 cups of curry.
5. Enjoy each serving with half of a piece of naan bread or 1 slice of crusty bread.

Nutrition:

- calories: 559; total fat: 16g; saturated fat: 7g; protein: 16g
- total carbs: 86g; fiber: 16g; sugar: 18g; sodium: 819mg

36. Stuffed Portobello with Cheese

Preparation Time: 15 minutes
Cooking Time: 25 minutes
Servings: 4
Ingredients:
- 4 Portobello mushroom caps
- 1 tablespoon olive oil
- 1/2 teaspoon salt, divided
- ¼ teaspoon freshly ground black pepper, divided
- 1 cup baby spinach, chopped
- 11/2 cups part-skim ricotta cheese
- 1/2 cup part-skim shredded mozzarella cheese

- ¼ cup grated parmesan cheese
- 1 garlic clove, minced
- 1 tablespoon dried parsley
- 2 teaspoons dried oregano
- 4 teaspoons unseasoned bread crumbs, divided
- 4 servings (4 cups) roasted broccoli with shallots

Directions:
1. Preheat the oven to 375f. Line a baking sheet with aluminum foil.
2. Brush the mushroom caps with the olive oil, and sprinkle with ¼ teaspoon salt and 1/8 teaspoon pepper. Put the mushroom caps on the prepared baking sheet and bake until soft, about 12 minutes.
3. In a medium bowl, mix the spinach, ricotta, mozzarella, parmesan, garlic, parsley, oregano, and the remaining ¼ teaspoon of salt 1/8 teaspoon of pepper.
4. Spoon 1/2 cup of cheese mixture into each mushroom cap, and sprinkle each with 1 teaspoon of bread crumbs. Return the mushrooms to the oven for an additional 8 to 10 minutes until warmed through.
5. Remove from the oven and allow the mushrooms to cool for about 10 minutes before placing each in an individual container. Add 1 cup of roasted broccoli with shallots to each container.

Nutrition:

- calories: 419; total fat: 30g
- saturated fat: 10g; protein: 23g
- total carbs: 19g; fiber: 2g
- sugar: 3g; sodium: 790mg

37. Lighter Shrimp Scampi

Preparation Time: 15 minutes
Cooking Time: 15 minutes
Servings: 4
Ingredients:
- 11/2 pounds large peeled and deveined shrimp
- ¼ teaspoon salt
- 1/8 teaspoon freshly ground black pepper

- 2 tablespoons olive oil
- 1 shallot, chopped
- 2 garlic cloves, minced
- ¼ cup cooking white wine
- Juice of 1/2 lemon (1 tablespoon)
- 1/2 teaspoon sriracha
- 2 tablespoons unsalted butter, at room temperature
- ¼ cup chopped fresh parsley
- 4 servings (6 cups) zucchini noodles with lemon vinaigrette

Directions:
1. Season the shrimp with the salt and pepper.
2. In a medium saucepan over medium heat, heat the oil. Add the shallot and garlic, and cook until the shallot softens and the garlic is fragrant, about 3 minutes. Add the shrimp, cover, and cook until opaque, 2 to 3 minutes on each side. Using a slotted spoon, transfer the shrimp to a large plate.
3. Add the wine, lemon juice, and sriracha to the saucepan, and stir to combine. Bring the mixture to a boil, then reduce the heat and simmer until the liquid is reduced by about half, 3 minutes. Add the butter and stir until melted, about 3 minutes. Return the shrimp to the saucepan and toss to coat. Add the parsley and stir to combine.
4. Into each of 4 containers, place 11/2 cups of zucchini noodles with lemon vinaigrette, and top with ¾ cup of scampi.

Nutrition:

- calories: 364; total fat: 21g; saturated fat: 6g; protein: 37g
- total carbs: 10g; fiber: 2g; sugar: 6g; sodium: 557mg

38. Maple-Mustard Salmon
Preparation Time: 10 minutes, plus 30 minutes marinating time
Cooking Time: 20 minutes
Servings: 4
Ingredients:
- Nonstick cooking spray
- 1/2 cup 100% maple syrup

- 2 tablespoons Dijon mustard
- ¼ teaspoon salt
- 4 (5-ounce) salmon fillets
- 4 servings (4 cups) roasted broccoli with shallots
- 4 servings (2 cups) parsleyed whole-wheat couscous

Directions:
1. Preheat the oven to 400f. Line a baking sheet with aluminum foil and coat with cooking spray.
2. In a medium bowl, whisk together the maple syrup, mustard, and salt until smooth.
3. Put the salmon fillets into the bowl and toss to coat. Cover and place in the refrigerator to marinate for at least 30 minutes and up to overnight.
4. Shake off excess marinade from the salmon fillets and place them on the prepared baking sheet, leaving a 1-inch space between each fillet. Discard the extra marinade.
5. Bake for about 20 minutes until the salmon is opaque. A thermometer inserted in the thickest part of a fillet reads 145f.
6. Into each of 4 resealable containers, place 1 salmon fillet, 1 cup of roasted broccoli with shallots, and 1/2 cup of parsleyed whole-wheat couscous.

Nutrition:

- calories: 601; total fat: 29g
- saturated fat: 4g; protein: 36g
- total carbs: 51g; fiber: 3g
- sugar: 23g; sodium: 610mg

39. Chicken Salad with Grapes and Pecans

Preparation Time: 15 Minutes
Cooking Time: 5 Minutes
Servings: 4
Ingredients:
- 1/3 cup unsalted pecans, chopped
- 10 ounces cooked skinless, boneless chicken breast or rotisserie chicken, finely chopped

- 1/2 medium yellow onion, finely chopped
- 1 celery stalk, finely chopped
- ¾ cup red or green seedless grapes, halved
- ¼ cup light mayonnaise
- ¼ cup nonfat plain Greek yogurt
- 1 tablespoon Dijon mustard
- 1 tablespoon dried parsley
- ¼ teaspoon salt
- 1/8 teaspoon freshly ground black pepper
- 1 cup shredded romaine lettuce
- 4 (8-inch) whole-wheat pitas

Directions:
1. Heat a small skillet over medium-low heat to toast the pecans. Cook the pecans until fragrant, about 3 minutes. Remove from the heat and set aside to cool.
2. In a medium bowl, mix the chicken, onion, celery, pecans, and grapes.
3. In a small bowl, whisk together the mayonnaise, yogurt, mustard, parsley, salt, and pepper. Spoon the sauce over the chicken mixture and stir until well combined.
4. Into each of 4 containers, place ¼ cup of lettuce and top with 1 cup of chicken salad. Store the pitas separately until ready to serve.
5. When ready to eat, stuff the serving of salad and lettuce into 1 pita.

Nutrition:
Calories: 418; Total Fat: 14g
Saturated Fat: 2g; Protein: 31g
Total Carbs: 43g; Fiber: 6g;

40. Roasted Vegetables
Preparation Time: 14 minutes
Cooking Time: 17 minutes
Servings: 3
Ingredients:
- 4 Tbsp. olive oil, reserve some for greasing

- 2 heads, large garlic, tops sliced off
- 2 large eggplants/aubergine, tops removed, cubed
- 2 large shallots, peeled, quartered
- 1 large carrot, peeled, cubed
- 1 large parsnips, peeled, cubed
- 1 small green bell pepper, deseeded, ribbed, cubed
- 1 small red bell pepper, deseeded, ribbed, cubed
- ½ pound Brussels sprouts, halved, do not remove cores
- 1 sprig, large thyme, leaves picked
- sea salt, coarse-grained

For garnish
- One large lemon halved, ½ squeezed, ½ sliced into smaller wedges
- 1/8 cup fennel bulb, minced

Directions:
1. From 425°F or 220°C preheat the oven for at least 5 minutes before using.
2. Line deep roasting pan with aluminum foil; lightly grease with oil. Tumble in bell peppers, Brussels sprouts, carrots, eggplants, garlic, parsnips, rosemary leaves, shallots, and thyme. Add a pinch of sea salt; drizzle in remaining oil and lemon juice. Toss well to combine.
3. Cover roasting pan with a sheet of aluminum foil. Place this on the middle rack of the oven. Bake for 20 to 30 minutes. Remove aluminum foil. Roast, for another 5 to 10 minutes, or until some vegetables brown at the edges. Remove roasting pan from oven. Cool slightly before spooning equal portions into plates.
4. Garnish with fennel and a wedge of lemon. Squeeze lemon juice on top of dish before eating.

Nutrition:

- Calories 163
- Total Fat 4.2 g
- Saturated Fat 0.8 g
- Cholesterol 0 mg
- Sodium 861 mg

- Total Carbs 22.5 g
- Fiber 6.3 g
- Sugar 2.3 g
- Protein 9.2 g

41. Millet Pilaf

Preparation Time: 10 minutes
Cooking Time: 15 minutes
Servings: 4
Ingredients:

- 1 cup millet
- 2 tomatoes, rinsed, seeded, and chopped
- 1¾ cups filtered water
- 2 tablespoons extra-virgin olive oil
- ¼ cup chopped dried apricot
- Zest of 1 lemon
- Juice of 1 lemon
- ½ cup fresh parsley, rinsed and chopped
- Himalayan pink salt
- Freshly ground black pepper

Directions:

1. In an electric pressure cooker, combine the millet, tomatoes, and water. Lock the lid into place, select Manual and High Pressure, and cook for 7 minutes.
2. When the beep sounds, quick release the pressure by pressing Cancel and twisting the steam valve to the Venting position. Carefully remove the lid.
3. Stir in the olive oil, apricot, lemon zest, lemon juice, and parsley. Taste, season with salt and pepper, and serve.

Nutrition:

- Calories: 270
- Total fat: 8g
- Total carbohydrates: 42g

- Fiber: 5g
- Sugar: 3g
- Protein: 6g

42. Sweet and Sour Onions

Preparation Time: 10 minutes
Cooking Time: 11 minutes
Servings: 4
Ingredients:
- 4 large onions, halved
- 2 garlic cloves, crushed
- 3 cups vegetable stock
- 1 ½ tablespoon balsamic vinegar
- ½ teaspoon Dijon mustard
- 1 tablespoon sugar

Directions:
1. Combine onions and garlic in a pan. Fry for 3 minutes, or till softened.
2. Pour stock, vinegar, Dijon mustard, and sugar. Bring to a boil.
3. Reduce heat. Cover and let the combination simmer for 10 minutes.
4. Get rid of from heat. Continue stirring until the liquid is reduced and the onions are brown. Serve.

Nutrition:

- Calories 203; Total Fat 41.2 g; Saturated Fat 0.8 g; Cholesterol 0 mg; Sodium 861 mg; Total Carbs 29.5 g; Fiber 16.3 g; Sugar 29.3 g; Protein 19.2 g

43. Sautéed Apples and Onions

Preparation Time: 14 minutes
Cooking Time: 16 minutes
Servings: 3

Ingredients:

- 2 cups dry cider
- 1 large onion, halved
- 2 cups vegetable stock
- 4 apples, sliced into wedges
- Pinch of salt
- Pinch of pepper

Directions:

1. Combine cider and onion in a saucepan. Bring to a boil until the onions are cooked and liquid almost gone.
2. Pour the stock and the apples. Season with salt and pepper. Stir occasionally. Cook for about 10 minutes or until the apples are tender but not mushy. Serve.

Nutrition:

- Calories 343
- Total Fat 51.2 g
- Saturated Fat 0.8 g
- Cholesterol 0 mg
- Sodium 861 mg
- Total Carbs 22.5 g
- Fiber 6.3 g
- Sugar 2.3 g
- Protein 9.2 g

44. Zucchini Noodles with Portabella Mushrooms

Preparation Time: 14 minutes
Cooking Time: 16 minutes
Servings: 3
Ingredients:

- 1 zucchini, processed into spaghetti-like noodles
- 3 garlic cloves, minced
- 2 white onions, thinly sliced
- 1 thumb-sized ginger, julienned
- 1 lb. chicken thighs
- 1 lb. portabella mushrooms, sliced into thick slivers

- 2 cups chicken stock
- 3 cups water
- Pinch of sea salt, add more if needed
- Pinch of black pepper, add more if needed
- 2 tsp. sesame oil
- 4 Tbsp. coconut oil, divided
- ¼ cup fresh chives, minced, for garnish

Directions:

1. Pour 2 tablespoons of coconut oil into a large saucepan. Fry mushroom slivers in batches for 5 minutes or until seared brown. Set aside. Transfer these to a plate.
2. Sauté the onion, garlic, and ginger for 3 minutes or until tender. Add in chicken thighs, cooked mushrooms, chicken stock, water, salt, and pepper stir mixture well. Bring to a boil.
3. Decrease gradually the heat and allow simmering for 20 minutes or until the chicken is forking tender. Tip in sesame oil.
4. Serve by placing an equal amount of zucchini noodles into bowls. Ladle soup and garnish with chives.

Nutrition:

- Calories 163
- Total Fat 4.2 g
- Saturated Fat 0.8 g
- Cholesterol 0 mg
- Sodium 861 mg
- Total Carbs 22.5 g
- Fiber 6.3 g
- Sugar 2.3 g, Protein 9.2 g

45. Grilled Tempeh with Pineapple

Preparation Time: 12 minutes
Cooking Time: 16 minutes
Servings: 3
Ingredients:

- 10 oz. tempeh, sliced
- 1 red bell pepper, quartered

- 1/4 pineapple, sliced into rings
- 6 oz. green beans
- 1 tbsp. coconut aminos
- 2 1/2 tbsp. orange juice, freshly squeeze
- 1 1/2 tbsp. lemon juice, freshly squeezed
- 1 tbsp. extra virgin olive oil
- 1/4 cup hoisin sauce

Directions:
1. Blend together the olive oil, orange and lemon juices, coconut aminos or soy sauce, and hoisin sauce in a bowl. Add the diced tempeh and set aside.
2. Heat up the grill or place a grill pan over medium high flame. Once hot, lift the marinated tempeh from the bowl with a pair of tongs and transfer them to the grill or pan.
3. Grille for 2 to 3 minutes, or until browned all over.
4. Grill the sliced pineapples alongside the tempeh, then transfer them directly onto the serving platter.
5. Place the grilled tempeh beside the grilled pineapple and cover with aluminum foil to keep warm.
6. Meanwhile, place the green beans and bell peppers in a bowl and add just enough of the marinade to coat.
7. Prepare the grill pan and add the vegetables. Grill until fork tender and slightly charred.
8. Transfer the grilled vegetables to the serving platter and arrange artfully with the tempeh and pineapple. Serve at once.

Nutrition:

- Calories 163;Total Fat 4.2 g; Saturated Fat 0.8 g; Cholesterol 0 mg
- Sodium 861 mg; Total Carbs 22.5 g; Fiber 6.3 g; Sugar 2.3 g; Protein 9.2 g

46. Courgettes In Cider Sauce

Preparation Time: 13 minutes
Cooking Time: 17 minutes
Servings: 3
Ingredients:

- 2 cups baby courgettes
- 3 tablespoons vegetable stock
- 2 tablespoons apple cider vinegar
- 1 tablespoon light brown sugar
- 4 spring onions, finely sliced
- 1-piece fresh gingerroot, grated
- 1 teaspoon corn flour
- 2 teaspoons water

Directions:

1. Bring a pan with salted water to a boil. Add courgettes. Bring to a boil for 5 minutes.
2. Meanwhile, in a pan, combine vegetable stock, apple cider vinegar, brown sugar, onions, gingerroot, lemon juice and rind, and orange juice and rind. Take to a boil. Lower the heat and allow simmering for 3 minutes.
3. Mix the corn flour with water. Stir well. Pour into the sauce. Continue stirring until the sauce thickens.
4. Drain courgettes. Transfer to the serving dish. Spoon over the sauce. Toss to coat courgettes. Serve.

Nutrition:

- Calories 173
- Total Fat 9.2 g
- Saturated Fat 0.8 g
- Cholesterol 0 mg
- Sodium 861 mg
- Total Carbs 22.5 g
- Fiber 6.3 g
- Sugar 2.3 g
- Protein 9.2 g

47. Baked Mixed Mushrooms

Preparation Time: 8 minutes
Cooking Time: 20 minutes
Servings: 3
Ingredients:

- 2 cups mixed wild mushrooms
- 1 cup chestnut mushrooms
- 2 cups dried porcini
- 2 shallots
- 4 garlic cloves
- 3 cups raw pecans
- ½ bunch fresh thyme
- 1 bunch flat-leaf parsley
- 2 tablespoons olive oil
- 2 fresh bay leaves
- 1 ½ cups stale bread

Directions:

1. Remove skin and finely chop garlic and shallots. Roughly chop the wild mushrooms and chestnut mushrooms. Pick the leaves of the thyme and tear the bread into small pieces. Put inside the pressure cooker.
2. Place the pecans and roughly chop the nuts. Pick the parsley leaves and roughly chop.
3. Place the porcini in a bowl then add 300ml of boiling water. Set aside until needed.
4. Heat oil in the pressure cooker. Add the garlic and shallots. Cook for 3 minutes while stirring occasionally.
5. Drain porcini and reserve the liquid. Add the porcini into the pressure cooker together with the wild mushrooms and chestnut mushrooms. Add the bay leaves and thyme.
6. Position the lid and lock in place. Put to high heat and bring to high pressure. Adjust heat to stabilize. Cook for 10 minutes. Adjust taste if necessary.
7. Transfer the mushroom mixture into a bowl and set aside to cool completely.
8. Once the mushrooms are completely cool, add the bread, pecans, a pinch of black pepper and sea salt, and half of the reserved liquid into the bowl. Mix well. Add more reserved liquid if the mixture seems dry.
9. Add more than half of the parsley into the bowl and stir. Transfer the mixture into a 20cm x 25cm lightly greased baking dish and cover with tin foil.

10. Bake in the oven for 35 minutes. Then, get rid of the foil and cook for another 10 minutes. Once done, sprinkle the remaining parsley on top and serve with bread or crackers. Serve.

Nutrition:

- Calories 343; Total Fat 4.2 g; Saturated Fat 0.8 g; Cholesterol 0 mg
- Sodium 861 mg; Total Carbs 22.5 g; Fiber 6.3 g; Sugar 2.3 g; Protein 9.2 g

48. Spiced Okra

Preparation Time: 14 minutes
Cooking Time: 16 minutes
Servings: 3
Ingredients:
- 2 cups okra
- ¼ teaspoon stevia
- 1 teaspoon chilli powder
- ½ teaspoon ground turmeric
- 1 tablespoon ground coriander
- 2 tablespoons fresh coriander, chopped
- 1 tablespoon ground cumin
- ¼ teaspoon salt
- 1 tablespoon desiccated coconut
- 3 tablespoons vegetable oil
- ½ teaspoon black mustard seeds
- ½ teaspoon cumin seeds
- Fresh tomatoes, to garnish

Directions:
1. Trim okra. Wash and dry.
2. Combine stevia, chilli powder, turmeric, ground coriander, fresh coriander, cumin, salt, and desiccated coconut in a bowl.
3. Heat the oil in a pan. Cook mustard and cumin seeds for 3 minutes. Stir continuously. Add okra. Tip in the spice mixture. Cook on low heat for 8 minutes.
4. Transfer to a serving dish. Garnish with fresh tomatoes.

Nutrition:

- Calories 163; Total Fat 4.2 g; Saturated Fat 0.8 g;Cholesterol 0 mg
- Sodium 861 mg; Total Carbs 22.5 g; Fiber 6.3 g; Sugar 2.3 g; Protein 9.2 g

Chapter 3.Dinner

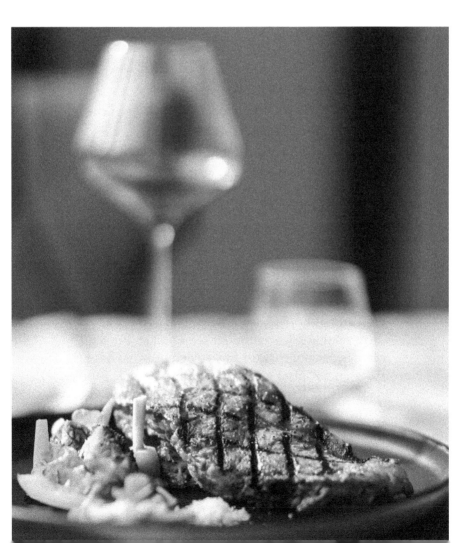

49. Cheesy Salmon Fillets

Preparation Time: 15 minutes
Cooking Time: 20 minutes
Servings: 2-3
Ingredients: For the salmon fillets

- 2 pieces, 4 oz. each salmon fillets, choose even cuts
- 1/2 cup sour cream, reduced fat
- ¼ cup cottage cheese, reduced fat
- ¼ cup Parmigiano-Reggiano cheese, freshly grated

Garnish:

- Spanish paprika
- 1/2 piece lemon, cut into wedges

Directions:

1. Preheat Air Fryer to 330 degrees F.
2. To make the salmon fillets, mix sour cream, cottage cheese, and Parmigiano-Reggiano cheese in a bowl.
3. Layer salmon fillets in the Air fryer basket. Fry for 20 minutes or until cheese turns golden brown.
4. To assemble, place a salmon fillet and sprinkle paprika. Garnish with lemon wedges and squeeze lemon juice on top. Serve.

Nutrition:

- Calorie: 274
- Carbohydrate: 1g
- Fat: 19g
- Protein: 24g; Fiber: 0.5g

50. Salmon with Asparagus

Preparation Time: 5 Minutes
Cooking Time: 10 Minutes
Servings: 3
Ingredients:

- 1 lb. Salmon, sliced into fillets
- 1 tbsp. Olive Oil
- Salt & Pepper, as needed
- 1 bunch of Asparagus, trimmed
- 2 cloves of Garlic, minced
- Zest & Juice of 1/2 Lemon
- 1 tbsp. Butter, salted

Directions:

1. Spoon in the butter and olive oil into a large pan and heat it over medium-high heat.
2. Once it becomes hot, place the salmon and season it with salt and pepper.
3. Cook for 4 minutes per side and then cook the other side.
4. Stir in the garlic and lemon zest to it.
5. Cook for further 2 minutes or until slightly browned.
6. Off the heat and squeeze the lemon juice over it.
7. Serve it hot.

Nutrition:

- Calories: 409Kcal
- Carbohydrates: 2.7g
- Proteins: 32.8g
- Fat: 28.8g
- Sodium: 497mg

51. Shrimp in Garlic Butter

Preparation Time: 5 Minutes
Cooking Time: 20 Minutes
Servings: 4
Ingredients:

- 1 lb. Shrimp, peeled & deveined
- ¼ tsp. Red Pepper Flakes
- 6 tbsp. Butter, divided
- 1/2 cup Chicken Stock
- Salt & Pepper, as needed
- 2 tbsp. Parsley, minced
- 5 cloves of Garlic, minced
- 2 tbsp. Lemon Juice

Directions:

1. Heat a large bottomed skillet over medium-high heat.
2. Spoon in two tablespoons of the butter and melt it. Add the shrimp.
3. Season it with salt and pepper. Sear for 4 minutes or until shrimp gets cooked.
4. Transfer the shrimp to a plate and stir in the garlic.
5. Sauté for 30 seconds or until aromatic.
6. Pour the chicken stock and whisk it well. Allow it to simmer for 5 to 10 minutes or until it has reduced to half.
7. Spoon the remaining butter, red pepper, and lemon juice to the sauce. Mix.
8. Continue cooking for another 2 minutes.
9. Take off the pan from the heat and add the cooked shrimp to it.
10. Garnish with parsley and transfer to the serving bowl.
11. Enjoy.

Nutrition:

- Calories: 307Kcal
- Carbohydrates: 3g
- Proteins: 27g
- Fat: 20g
- Sodium: 522mg

52. Cobb Salad

Keto & Under 30 Minutes
Preparation Time: 5 Minutes
Cooking Time: 5 Minutes
Servings: 1
Ingredients:

- 4 Cherry Tomatoes, chopped
- ¼ cup Bacon, cooked & crumbled
- 1/2 of 1 Avocado, chopped
- 2 oz. Chicken Breast, shredded
- 1 Egg, hardboiled
- 2 cups Mixed Green salad
- 1 oz. Feta Cheese, crumbled

Directions:

1. Toss all the **Ingredients** for the Cobb salad in a large mixing bowl and toss well.
2. Serve and enjoy it.

Nutrition:

- Calories: 307Kcal
- Carbohydrates: 3g
- Proteins: 27g
- Fat: 20g
- Sodium: 522mg

53. Seared Tuna Steak

Preparation Time: 10 Minutes
Cooking Time: 10 Minutes
Serving Size: 2
Ingredients:

- 1 tsp. Sesame Seeds
- 1 tbsp. Sesame Oil
- 2 tbsp. Soya Sauce
- Salt & Pepper, to taste
- 2 × 6 oz. Ahi Tuna Steaks

Directions:
1. Seasoning the tuna steaks with salt and pepper. Keep it aside on a shallow bowl.
2. In another bowl, mix soya sauce and sesame oil.
3. pour the sauce over the salmon and coat them generously with the sauce.
4. Keep it aside for 10 to 15 minutes and then heat a large skillet over medium heat.
5. Once hot, keep the tuna steaks and cook them for 3 minutes or until seared underneath.
6. Flip the fillets and cook them for a further 3 minutes.
7. Transfer the seared tuna steaks to the serving plate and slice them into 1/2 inch slices. Top with sesame seeds.

Nutrition:

- Calories: 255Kcal
- Fat: 9g
- Carbohydrates: 1g
- Proteins: 40.5g; Sodium: 293mg

54. Beef Chili

Preparation Time: 10 Minutes
Cooking Time: 20 Minutes
Serving Size: 4
Ingredients:
- 1/2 tsp. Garlic Powder
- 1 tsp. Coriander, grounded
- 1 lb. Beef, grounded
- 1/2 tsp. Sea Salt
- 1/2 tsp. Cayenne Pepper
- 1 tsp. Cumin, grounded
- 1/2 tsp. Pepper, grounded
- 1/2 cup Salsa, low-carb & no-sugar

Directions:
1. Heat a large-sized pan over medium-high heat and cook the beef in it until browned.

2. Stir in all the spices and cook them for 7 minutes or until everything is combined.
3. When the beef gets cooked, spoon in the salsa.
4. Bring the mixture to a simmer and cook for another 8 minutes or until everything comes together.
5. Take it from heat and transfer to a serving bowl.

Nutrition:

- Calories: 229Kcal
- Fat: 10g
- Carbohydrates: 2g
- Proteins: 33g; Sodium: 675mg

55. Greek Broccoli Salad

Preparation Time: 10 Minutes
Cooking Time: 15 Minutes
Servings: 4
Ingredients:

- 1 ¼ lb. Broccoli, sliced into small bites
- ¼ cup Almonds, sliced
- 1/3 cup Sun-dried Tomatoes
- ¼ cup Feta Cheese, crumbled
- ¼ cup Red Onion, sliced

For the dressing:

- 1/4 cup Olive Oil
- Dash of Red Pepper Flakes
- 1 Garlic clove, minced
- ¼ tsp. Salt
- 2 tbsp. Lemon Juice
- 1/2 tsp. Dijon Mustard
- 1 tsp. Low Carb Sweetener Syrup
- 1/2 tsp. Oregano, dried

Directions:

1. Mix broccoli, onion, almonds and sun-dried tomatoes in a large mixing bowl.

2. In another small-sized bowl, combine all the dressing **Ingredients** until emulsified.
3. Spoon the dressing over the broccoli salad.
4. Allow the salad to rest for half an hour before serving.

Nutrition:

- Calories: 272Kcal
- Carbohydrates: 11.9g
- Proteins: 8g
- Fat: 21.6g
- Sodium: 321mg

56. Cold Cauliflower-Coconut Soup

Preparation Time: 7 minutes
Cooking Time: 20 minutes
Servings: 3-4
Ingredients:
- 1 pound (450g) new cauliflower
- 1 ¼ cup (300ml) unsweetened coconut milk
- 1 cup water (best: antacid water)
- 2 tbsp. new lime juice
- 1/3 cup cold squeezed additional virgin olive oil
- 1 cup new coriander leaves, slashed
- Spot of salt and cayenne pepper
- 1 bunch of unsweetened coconut chips

Directions:
1. Steam cauliflower for around 10 minutes.
2. At that point, set up the cauliflower with coconut milk and water in a food processor and procedure until extremely smooth.
3. Include new lime squeeze, salt and pepper, a large portion of the cleaved coriander and the oil and blend for an additional couple of moments.
4. Pour in soup bowls and embellishment with coriander and coconut chips. Appreciate!

Nutrition:

- Calories: 65, Carbohydrates: 11g
- Fat: 0.3g, Protein: 1.5g

57. Raw Avocado-Broccoli Soup with Cashew Nuts

Preparation Time: 10 minutes
Cooking Time: 30 minutes
Servings: 1-2
Ingredients:
- ½ cup water (if available: alkaline water)
- ½ avocado
- 1 cup chopped broccoli
- ½ cup cashew nuts
- ½ cup alfalfa sprouts
- 1 clove of garlic
- 1 tbsp. cold pressed extra virgin olive oil
- 1 pinch of sea salt and pepper
- Some parsley to garnish

Directions:
1. Put the cashew nuts in a blender or food processor, include some water and puree for a couple of moments.
2. Include the various fixings (with the exception of the avocado) individually and puree each an ideal opportunity for a couple of moments.
3. Dispense the soup in a container and warm it up to the normal room temperature. Enhance with salt and pepper. In the interim dice the avocado and slash the parsley.
4. Dispense the soup in a container or plate; include the avocado dices and embellishment with parsley.
5. That's it! Enjoy this excellent healthy soup!

Nutrition:

- Calories: 48
- Carbohydrates: 18g
- Fat: 3g
- Protein: 1.4g

58. Quick Broccoli Soup

Preparation Time: 5 minutes
Cooking Time: 10 minutes
Servings: 6
Ingredients:

- 1 lb. broccoli, chopped
- 6 cups filtered alkaline water
- 1 onion, diced
- 2 tbsp. olive oil
- Pepper
- Salt

Directions:

1. Add oil into the instant pot and set the pot on sauté mode.
2. Add onion in olive oil and sauté until softened.
3. Add broccoli and water and stir well.
4. Cover pot with top and cook on manual high pressure for 3 minutes.
5. When finished, release pressure using the quick release **Directions:** than open the lid.
6. Blend the soup utilizing a submersion blender until smooth.
7. Season soup with pepper and salt.
8. Serve and enjoy.

Nutrition:

- Calories 73
- Fat 4.9 g
- Carbohydrates 6.7 g
- Protein 2.3 g
- Sugar 2.1 g; Cholesterol 0 mg

59. Green Lentil Soup

Preparation Time: 10 minutes
Cooking Time: 30 minutes
Servings: 4
Ingredients:

- 1 ½ cups green lentils, rinsed

- 4 cups baby spinach
- 4 cups filtered alkaline water
- 1 tsp. Italian seasoning
- 2 tsp. fresh thyme
- 14 oz. tomatoes, diced
- 3 garlic cloves, minced
- 2 celery stalks, chopped
- 1 carrot, chopped
- 1 onion, chopped
- Pepper
- Sea salt

Directions:
1. Add all **Ingredients** except spinach into the direct pot and mix fine.
2. Cover pot with top and cook on manual high pressure for 18 minutes.
3. When finished, release pressure using the quick release **Directions:** than open the lid.
4. Add spinach and stir well.
5. Serve and enjoy.

Nutrition:

- Calories 306
- Fat 1.5 g
- Carbohydrates 53.7 g
- Sugar 6.4 g
- Protein 21 g
- Cholesterol 1 mg

60. Squash Soup

Preparation Time: 10 minutes
Cooking Time: 40 minutes
Servings: 4
Ingredients:
- 3 lbs. butternut squash, peeled and cubed
- 1 tbsp. curry powder

- 1/2 cup unsweetened coconut milk
- 3 cups filtered alkaline water
- 2 garlic cloves, minced
- 1 large onion, minced
- 1 tsp. olive oil

Directions:
1. Add olive oil in the instant pot and set the pot on sauté mode.
2. Add onion and cook until tender, about 8 minutes.
3. Add curry powder and garlic and sauté for a minute.
4. Add butternut squash, water, and salt and stir well.
5. Cover pot with lid and cook on soup mode for 30 minutes.
6. When finished, allow to release pressure naturally for 10 minutes then release using quick release **Directions:** than open the lid.
7. Blend the soup utilizing a submersion blender until smooth.
8. Add coconut milk and stir well.
9. Serve warm and enjoy.

Nutrition:

- Calories 254
- Fat 8.9 g
- Carbohydrates 46.4 g
- Sugar 10.1 g
- Protein 4.8 g
- Cholesterol 0 mg

61. Tomato Soup

Preparation Time: 5 minutes
Cooking Time: 20 minutes
Servings: 4
Ingredients:
- 6 tomatoes, chopped
- 1 onion, diced
- 14 oz. coconut milk
- 1 tsp. turmeric
- 1 tsp. garlic, minced
- 1/4 cup cilantro, chopped

- 1/2 tsp. cayenne pepper
- 1 tsp. ginger, minced
- 1/2 tsp. sea salt

Directions:
1. Add all **Ingredients** to the direct pot and mix fine.
2. Cover instant pot with lid and cook on manual high pressure for 5 minutes.
3. When finished, allow to release pressure naturally for 10 minutes then release using the quick release **Directions**:
4. Blend the soup utilizing a submersion blender until smooth.
5. Stir well and serve.

Nutrition:

- Calories 81
- Fat 3.5 g
- Carbohydrates 11.6 g
- Sugar 6.1 g
- Protein 2.5 g
- Cholesterol 0 mg

62. Basil Zucchini Soup

Preparation Time: 10 minutes
Cooking Time: 20 minutes
Servings: 4
Ingredients:
- 3 medium zucchinis, peeled and chopped
- 1/4 cup basil, chopped
- 1 large leek, chopped
- 3 cups filtered alkaline water
- 1 tbsp. lemon juice
- 3 tbsp. olive oil
- 2 tsp. sea salt

Directions:
1. Add 2 tbsp. oil into the pot and set the pot on sauté mode.
2. Add zucchini and sauté for 5 minutes.

3. Add basil and leeks and sauté for 2-3 minutes.
4. Add lemon juice, water, and salt. Stir well.
5. Cover pot with lid and cook on high pressure for 8 minutes.
6. When finished, allow to release pressure naturally then open the lid.
7. Blend the soup utilizing a submersion blender until smooth.
8. Top with remaining olive oil and serve.

Nutrition:

- Calories 157; Fat 11.9 g; Carbohydrates 8.9 g
- Protein 5.8 gSugar 4 g; Cholesterol 0 mg

63. Summer Vegetable Soup

Preparation Time: 5 minutes
Cooking Time: 20 minutes
Servings: 10
Ingredients:
- 1/2 cup basil, chopped
- 2 bell peppers, seeded and sliced
- 1/ cup green beans, trimmed and cut into pieces
- 8 cups filtered alkaline water
- 1 medium summer squash, sliced
- 1 medium zucchini, sliced
- 2 large tomatoes, sliced
- 1 small eggplant, sliced
- 6 garlic cloves, smashed
- 1 medium onion, diced
- Pepper
- Salt

Directions:
1. Combine all elements into the direct pot and mix fine.
2. Cover pot with lid and cook on soup mode for 10 minutes.
3. Release pressure using quick release **Directions:** than open the lid.
4. Blend the soup utilizing a submersion blender until smooth.
5. Serve and enjoy.

Nutrition:

- Calories 84
- Fat 1.6 g
- Carbohydrates 12.8 g
- Protein 6.1 g
- Sugar 6.1 g
- Cholesterol 0 mg

64. Swordfish Steak

Preparation Time: 10 minutes
Cooking Time: 35 Minutes
Servings: 2
Ingredients:

- 1lb swordfish steak, whole
- 1lb chopped Mediterranean vegetables
- 1 cup low sodium fish broth
- 2tbsp soy sauce

Directions:

1. Mix all the **Ingredients** except the broth in a foil pouch.
2. Place the pouch in the steamer basket for your Instant Pot.
3. Pour the broth into the Instant Pot. Lower the steamer basket into the Instant Pot.
4. Cook on Steam for 35 minutes.
5. Release the pressure naturally.

Nutrition:

- Calories: 270
- Carbs: 5
- Sugar: 1
- Fat: 10
- Protein: 48

- GL: 1

65. Lemon Sole

Preparation Time: 10 minutes
Cooking Time: 5 Minutes
Servings: 2
Ingredients:
- 1lb sole fillets, boned and skinned
- 1 cup low sodium fish broth
- 2 shredded sweet onions
- juice of half a lemon
- 2tbsp dried cilantro

Directions:
1. Mix all the **Ingredients** in your Instant Pot.
2. Cook on Stew for 5 minutes.
3. Release the pressure naturally.

Nutrition:

- Calories: 230
- Sugar: 1
- Fat: 6
- Protein: 46
- GL: 1

66. Cheesy Cauliflower Gratin

Preparation Time: 5 Minutes
Cooking Time: 25 Minutes
Servings: 6
Ingredients:
- 6 deli slices Pepper Jack Cheese
- 4 cups Cauliflower florets
- Salt and Pepper, as needed
- 4 tbsp. Butter
- 1/3 cup Heavy Whipping Cream

Directions:

1. Mix the cauliflower, cream, butter, salt, and pepper in a safe microwave bowl and combine well.
2. Microwave the cauliflower mixture for 25 minutes on high until it becomes soft and tender.
3. Remove the ingredients from the bowl and mash with the help of a fork.
4. Taste for seasonings and spoon in salt and pepper as required.
5. Arrange the slices of pepper jack cheese on top of the cauliflower mixture and microwave for 3 minutes until the cheese starts melting.
6. Serve warm.

Nutrition:

- Calories: 421Kcal
- Carbohydrates: 3g
- Proteins: 19g
- Fat: 37g
- Sodium: 111mg

67. Strawberry Spinach Salad

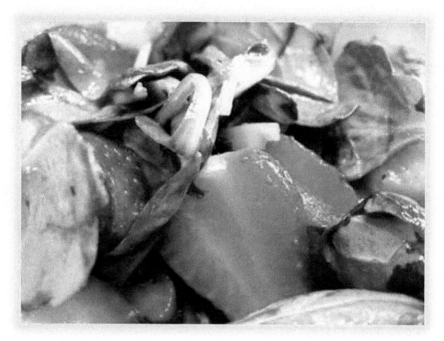

Preparation Time: 5 Minutes
Cooking Time: 10 Minutes
Servings: 4
Ingredients:

- 4 oz. Feta Cheese, crumbled
- 8 Strawberries, sliced
- 2 oz. Almonds
- 6 Slices Bacon, thick-cut, crispy and crumbled
- 10 oz. Spinach leaves, fresh
- 2 Roma Tomatoes, diced
- 2 oz. Red Onion, sliced thinly

Directions:

1. For making this healthy salad, mix all the ingredients needed to make the salad in a large-sized bowl and toss them well.

Nutrition:

- Calories – 255kcal
- Fat – 16g

- Carbohydrates – 8g
- Proteins – 14g
- Sodium: 27mg

68. Cauliflower Mac & Cheese

Preparation Time: 5 Minutes
Cooking Time: 25 Minutes
Effort: Easy
Serving Size: 4
Ingredients:

- 1 Cauliflower Head, torn into florets
- Salt & Black Pepper, as needed
- ¼ cup Almond Milk, unsweetened
- ¼ cup Heavy Cream
- 3 tbsp. Butter, preferably grass-fed
- 1 cup Cheddar Cheese, shredded

Directions:

1. Preheat the oven to 450 F.
2. Melt the butter in a small microwave-safe bowl and heat it for 30 seconds.
3. Pour the melted butter over the cauliflower florets along with salt and pepper. Toss them well.
4. Place the cauliflower florets in a parchment paper-covered large baking sheet.
5. Bake them for 15 minutes or until the cauliflower is crisp-tender.

6. Once baked, mix the heavy cream, cheddar cheese, almond milk, and the remaining butter in a large microwave-safe bowl and heat it on high heat for 2 minutes or until the cheese mixture is smooth. Repeat the procedure until the cheese has melted.
7. Finally, stir in the cauliflower to the sauce mixture and coat well.

Nutrition:

- Calories: 294Kcal
- Fat: 23g
- Carbohydrates: 7g
- Proteins: 11g

69. Easy Egg Salad

Preparation Time: 5 Minutes
Cooking Time: 15 to 20 Minutes
Effort: Easy
Servings: 4
Ingredients:

- 6 Eggs, preferably free-range
- ¼ tsp. Salt
- 2 tbsp. Mayonnaise
- 1 tsp. Lemon juice
- 1 tsp. Dijon mustard
- Pepper, to taste
- Lettuce leaves, to serve

Directions:

1. Keep the eggs in a saucepan of water and pour cold water until it covers the egg by another 1 inch.
2. Bring to a boil and then remove the eggs from heat.
3. Peel the eggs under cold running water.
4. Transfer the cooked eggs into a food processor and pulse them until chopped.
5. Stir in the mayonnaise, lemon juice, salt, Dijon mustard, and pepper and mix them well.
6. Taste for seasoning and add more if required.
7. Serve in the lettuce leaves.

Nutrition:

- Calories – 166kcal
- Fat – 14g
- Carbohydrates - 0.85g
- Proteins – 10g

70. Baked Chicken Legs

Preparation Time: 10 Minutes
Cooking Time: 40 Minutes
Effort: Easy
Servings: 6
Ingredients:
- 6 Chicken Legs
- ¼ tsp. Black Pepper
- ¼ cup Butter
- 1/2 tsp. Sea Salt
- 1/2 tsp. Smoked Paprika
- 1/2 tsp. Garlic Powder

Directions:
1. Preheat the oven to 425 F.
2. Pat the chicken legs with a paper towel to absorb any excess moisture.
3. Marinate the chicken pieces by first applying the butter over them and then with the seasoning. Set it aside for a few minutes.
4. Bake them for 25 minutes. Turnover and bake for further 10 minutes or until the internal temperature reaches 165 F.
5. Serve them hot.

Nutrition:

- Calories – 236kL
- Fat – 16g
- Carbohydrates – 0g
- Protein – 22g
- Sodium – 314mg

71. Creamed Spinach

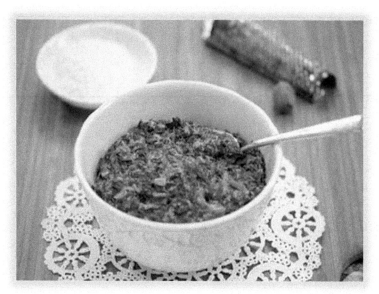

Preparation Time: 5 Minutes
Cooking Time: 10 Minutes
Effort: Easy
Servings: 4
Ingredients:

- 3 tbsp. Butter
- ¼ tsp. Black Pepper
- 4 cloves of Garlic, minced
- ¼ tsp. Sea Salt
- 10 oz. Baby Spinach, chopped
- 1 tsp. Italian Seasoning
- 1/2 cup Heavy Cream
- 3 oz. Cream Cheese

Directions:

1. Melt butter in a large sauté pan over medium heat.
2. Once the butter has melted, spoon in the garlic and sauté for 3o seconds or until aromatic.
3. Spoon in the spinach and cook for 3 to 4 minutes or until wilted.
4. Add all the remaining ingredients to it and continuously stir until the cream cheese melts and the mixture gets thickened.
5. Serve hot

Nutrition:

- Calories – 274kL
- Fat – 27g
- Carbohydrates – 4g
- Protein – 4g
- Sodium – 114mg

72. Stuffed Mushrooms

Preparation Time: 10 Minutes
Cooking Time: 20 Minutes
Servings: 4
Ingredients:

- 4 Portobello Mushrooms, large
- 1/2 cup Mozzarella Cheese, shredded
- 1/2 cup Marinara, low-sugar
- Olive Oil Spray

Directions:

1. Preheat the oven to 375 F.
2. Take out the dark gills from the mushrooms with the help of a spoon.
3. Keep the mushroom stem upside down and spoon it with two tablespoons of marinara sauce and mozzarella cheese.
4. Bake for 18 minutes or until the cheese is bubbly.

Nutrition:

- Calories – 113kL
- Fat – 6g
- Carbohydrates – 4g
- Protein – 7g
- Sodium – 14mg

73. Vegetable Soup

Preparation Time: 10 Minutes
Cooking Time: 30 Minutes
Servings: 5
Ingredients:

- 8 cups Vegetable Broth
- 2 tbsp. Olive Oil
- 1 tbsp. Italian Seasoning
- 1 Onion, large & diced
- 2 Bay Leaves, dried
- 2 Bell Pepper, large & diced
- Sea Salt & Black Pepper, as needed
- 4 cloves of Garlic, minced
- 28 oz. Tomatoes, diced
- 1 Cauliflower head, medium & torn into florets
- 2 cups Green Beans, trimmed & chopped

Directions:

1. Heat oil in a Dutch oven over medium heat.
2. Once the oil becomes hot, stir in the onions and pepper.
3. Cook for 10 minutes or until the onion is softened and browned.
4. Spoon in the garlic and sauté for a minute or until fragrant.
5. Add all the remaining ingredients to it. Mix until everything comes together.
6. Bring the mixture to a boil. Lower the heat and cook for further 20 minutes or until the vegetables have softened.
7. Serve hot.

Nutrition:

- Calories – 79kL
- Fat – 2g
- Carbohydrates – 8g
- Protein – 2g
- Sodium – 187mg

74. Pork Chop Diane

Preparation Time: 10 minutes
Cooking Time: 20 minutes
Serving: 4
Ingredients:

- ¼ cup low-sodium chicken broth
- 1 tablespoon freshly squeezed lemon juice
- 2 teaspoons Worcestershire sauce
- 2 teaspoons Dijon mustard
- 4 (5-ounce) boneless pork top loin chops
- 1 teaspoon extra-virgin olive oil
- 1 teaspoon lemon zest
- 1 teaspoon butter
- 2 teaspoons chopped fresh chives

Direction:

1. Blend together the chicken broth, lemon juice, Worcestershire sauce, and Dijon mustard and set it aside.
2. Season the pork chops lightly.
3. Situate large skillet over medium-high heat and add the olive oil.
4. Cook the pork chops, turning once, until they are no longer pink, about 8 minutes per side.
5. Put aside the chops.
6. Pour the broth mixture into the skillet and cook until warmed through and thickened, about 2 minutes.
7. Blend lemon zest, butter, and chives.
8. Garnish with a generous spoonful of sauce.

Nutrition:

- 200 Calories
- 8g Fat
- 1g Carbohydrates

75. Autumn Pork Chops with Red Cabbage and Apples

Preparation Time: 15 minutes
Cooking Time: 30 minutes

Serving: 4
Ingredients:

- ¼ cup apple cider vinegar
- 2 tablespoons granulated sweetener
- 4 (4-ounce) pork chops, about 1 inch thick
- 1 tablespoon extra-virgin olive oil
- ½ red cabbage, finely shredded
- 1 sweet onion, thinly sliced
- 1 apple, peeled, cored, and sliced
- 1 teaspoon chopped fresh thyme

Direction:

1. Scourge together the vinegar and sweetener. Set it aside.
2. Season the pork with salt and pepper.
3. Position huge skillet over medium-high heat and add the olive oil.
4. Cook the pork chops until no longer pink, turning once, about 8 minutes per side.
5. Put chops aside.
6. Add the cabbage and onion to the skillet and sauté until the vegetables have softened, about 5 minutes.
7. Add the vinegar mixture and the apple slices to the skillet and bring the mixture to a boil.
8. Adjust heat to low and simmer, covered, for 5 additional minutes.
9. Return the pork chops to the skillet, along with any accumulated juices and thyme, cover, and cook for 5 more minutes.

Nutrition:

- 223 Calories
- 12g Carbohydrates
- 3g Fiber

76. Chipotle Chili Pork Chops

Preparation Time: 4 hours
Cooking Time: 20 minutes
Serving: 4
Ingredients:

- Juice and zest of 1 lime
- 1 tablespoon extra-virgin olive oil
- 1 tablespoon chipotle chili powder
- 2 teaspoons minced garlic
- 1 teaspoon ground cinnamon
- Pinch sea salt
- 4 (5-ounce) pork chops

Direction:

1. Combine the lime juice and zest, oil, chipotle chili powder, garlic, cinnamon, and salt in a resealable plastic bag. Add the pork chops. Remove as much air as possible and seal the bag.
2. Marinate the chops in the refrigerator for at least 4 hours, and up to 24 hours, turning them several times.
3. Ready the oven to 400°F and set a rack on a baking sheet. Let the chops rest at room temperature for 15 minutes, then arrange them on the rack and discard the remaining marinade.
4. Roast the chops until cooked through, turning once, about 10 minutes per side.
5. Serve with lime wedges.

Nutrition:

- 204 Calories
- 1g Carbohydrates
- 1g Sugar

77. Orange-Marinated Pork Tenderloin

Preparation Time: 2 hours
Cooking Time: 30 minutes
Serving: 4
Ingredients:

- ¼ cup freshly squeezed orange juice

- 2 teaspoons orange zest
- 2 teaspoons minced garlic
- 1 teaspoon low-sodium soy sauce
- 1 teaspoon grated fresh ginger
- 1 teaspoon honey
- 1½ pounds pork tenderloin roast
- 1 tablespoon extra-virgin olive oil

Direction:

1. Blend together the orange juice, zest, garlic, soy sauce, ginger, and honey.
2. Pour the marinade into a resealable plastic bag and add the pork tenderloin.
3. Remove as much air as possible and seal the bag. Marinate the pork in the refrigerator, turning the bag a few times, for 2 hours.
4. Preheat the oven to 400°F.
5. Pull out tenderloin from the marinade and discard the marinade.
6. Position big ovenproof skillet over medium-high heat and add the oil.
7. Sear the pork tenderloin on all sides, about 5 minutes in total.
8. Position skillet to the oven and roast for 25 minutes.
9. Put aside for 10 minutes before serving.

Nutrition:

- 228 Calories
- 4g Carbohydrates
- 3g Sugar

78. Homestyle Herb Meatballs

Preparation Time: 10 minutes
Cooking Time: 15 minutes
Serving: 4
Ingredients:
- ½ pound lean ground pork

- ½ pound lean ground beef
- 1 sweet onion, finely chopped
- ¼ cup bread crumbs
- 2 tablespoons chopped fresh basil
- 2 teaspoons minced garlic
- 1 egg

Direction:

1. Preheat the oven to 350°F.
2. Ready baking tray with parchment paper and set it aside.
3. In a large bowl, mix together the pork, beef, onion, bread crumbs, basil, garlic, egg, salt, and pepper until very well mixed.
4. Roll the meat mixture into 2-inch meatballs.
5. Transfer the meatballs to the baking sheet and bake until they are browned and cooked through, about 15 minutes.
6. Serve the meatballs with your favorite marinara sauce and some steamed green beans.

Nutrition:

- 332 Calories
- 13g Carbohydrates
- 3g Sugar

79. Lime-Parsley Lamb Cutlets

Preparation Time: 4 hours
Cooking Time: 10 minutes
Serving: 4
Ingredients:

- ¼ cup extra-virgin olive oil
- ¼ cup freshly squeezed lime juice
- 2 tablespoons lime zest
- 2 tablespoons chopped fresh parsley
- 12 lamb cutlets (about 1½ pounds total)

Direction:

1. Scourge the oil, lime juice, zest, parsley, salt, and pepper.

2. Pour marinade to a resealable plastic bag.
3. Add the cutlets to the bag and remove as much air as possible before sealing.
4. Marinate the lamb in the refrigerator for about 4 hours, turning the bag several times.
5. Preheat the oven to broil.
6. Remove the chops from the bag and arrange them on an aluminum foil–lined baking sheet. Discard the marinade.
7. Broil the chops for 4 minutes per side for medium doneness.
8. Let the chops rest for 5 minutes before serving.

Nutrition:

- 413 Calories
- 1g Carbohydrates
- 31g Protein

80. Mediterranean Steak Sandwiches

Preparation Time: 1 hour
Cooking Time: 10 minutes
Serving: 4
Ingredients:

- 2 tablespoons extra-virgin olive oil
- 2 tablespoons balsamic vinegar
- 2 teaspoons garlic
- 2 teaspoons lemon juice
- 2 teaspoons fresh oregano
- 1 teaspoon fresh parsley
- 1-pound flank steak
- 4 whole-wheat pitas
- 2 cups shredded lettuce
- 1 red onion, thinly sliced
- 1 tomato, chopped
- 1 ounce low-sodium feta cheese

Direction:

1. Scourge olive oil, balsamic vinegar, garlic, lemon juice, oregano, and parsley.

2. Add the steak to the bowl, turning to coat it completely.
3. Marinate the steak for 1 hour in the refrigerator, turning it over several times.
4. Preheat the broiler. Line a baking sheet with aluminum foil.
5. Put steak out of the bowl and discard the marinade.
6. Situate steak on the baking sheet and broil for 5 minutes per side for medium.
7. Set aside for 10 minutes before slicing.
8. Stuff the pitas with the sliced steak, lettuce, onion, tomato, and feta.

Nutrition:

- 344 Calories
- 22g Carbohydrates
- 3g Fiber

81. Roasted Beef with Peppercorn Sauce

Preparation Time: 10 minutes
Cooking Time: 90 minutes
Serving: 4
Ingredients:

- 1½ pounds top rump beef roast
- 3 teaspoons extra-virgin olive oil
- 3 shallots, minced
- 2 teaspoons minced garlic
- 1 tablespoon green peppercorns
- 2 tablespoons dry sherry
- 2 tablespoons all-purpose flour
- 1 cup sodium-free beef broth

Direction:

1. Heat the oven to 300°F.
2. Season the roast with salt and pepper.
3. Position huge skillet over medium-high heat and add 2 teaspoons of olive oil.
4. Brown the beef on all sides, about 10 minutes in total, and transfer the roast to a baking dish.

5. Roast until desired doneness, about 1½ hours for medium. When the roast has been in the oven for 1 hour, start the sauce.
6. In a medium saucepan over medium-high heat, sauté the shallots in the remaining 1 teaspoon of olive oil until translucent, about 4 minutes.
7. Stir in the garlic and peppercorns, and cook for another minute. Whisk in the sherry to deglaze the pan.
8. Whisk in the flour to form a thick paste, cooking for 1 minute and stirring constantly.
9. Fill in the beef broth and whisk for 4 minutes. Season the sauce.
10. Serve the beef with a generous spoonful of sauce.

Nutrition:

- 330 Calories
- 4g Carbohydrates
- 36g Protein

Chapter 4.Dessert and Sweets

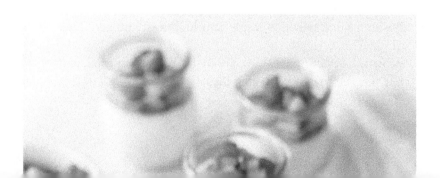

82. Fruit Pizza

Preparation Time: 5 minutes
Cooking Time: 10 minutes
Servings: 4
Ingredients:
- 1 teaspoon maple syrup

- ¼ teaspoon vanilla extract
- ½ cup coconut milk yogurt
- 2 round slices watermelon
- ½ cup blackberries, sliced
- ½ cup strawberries, sliced
- 2 tablespoons coconut flakes (unsweetened)

Directions:

1. Mix maple syrup, vanilla and yogurt in a bowl.
2. Spread the mixture on top of the watermelon slice.
3. Top with the berries and coconut flakes.

Nutrition:

- 70 Calories
- 14.6g Carbohydrate
- 1.2g Protein

83. Choco Peppermint Cake

Preparation Time: 5 minutes
Cooking Time: 10 minutes
Servings: 4
Ingredients:

- Cooking spray
- 1/3 cup oil
- 15 oz. package chocolate cake mix
- 3 eggs, beaten
- 1 cup water
- ¼ teaspoon peppermint extract

Directions:

1. Spray slow cooker with oil.
2. Mix all the **Ingredients** in a bowl.
3. Use an electric mixer on medium speed setting to mix **Ingredients** for 2 minutes.
4. Pour mixture into the slow cooker.

5. Cover the pot and cook on low for 3 hours.
6. Let cool before slicing and serving.

Nutrition:

- 185 Calories
- 27g Carbohydrate
- 3.8g Protein

84. Roasted Mango

Preparation Time: 5 minutes
Cooking Time: 10 minutes
Servings: 4
Ingredients:

- 2 mangoes, sliced
- 2 teaspoons crystallized ginger, chopped
- 2 teaspoons orange zest
- 2 tablespoons coconut flakes (unsweetened)

Directions:

1. Preheat your oven to 350 degrees F.
2. Add mango slices in custard cups.
3. Top with the ginger, orange zest and coconut flakes.
4. Bake in the oven for 10 minutes.

Nutrition:

- 89 Calories
- 20g Carbohydrate
- 0.8g Protein

85. Roasted Plums

Preparation Time: 5 minutes
Cooking Time: 10 minutes
Servings: 4
Ingredients:

- Cooking spray

- 6 plums, sliced
- ½ cup pineapple juice (unsweetened)
- 1 tablespoon brown sugar
- 2 tablespoons brown sugar
- ¼ teaspoon ground cardamom
- ½ teaspoon ground cinnamon
- 1/8 teaspoon ground cumin

Directions:

1. Combine all the **Ingredients** in a baking pan.
2. Roast in the oven at 450 degrees F for 20 minutes.

Nutrition:

- 102 Calories
- 18.7g Carbohydrate
- 2g Protein

86. Figs with Honey & Yogurt

Preparation Time: 5 minutes
Cooking Time: 10 minutes
Servings: 4
Ingredients:

- ½ teaspoon vanilla
- 8 oz. nonfat yogurt
- 2 figs, sliced
- 1 tablespoon walnuts, chopped and toasted
- 2 teaspoons honey

Directions:

1. Stir vanilla into yogurt.
2. Mix well.
3. Top with the figs and sprinkle with walnuts.
4. Drizzle with honey and serve.

Nutrition:

- 157 Calories
- 24g Carbohydrate
- 7g Protein

87. Butternut Squash Pie

Preparation Time: 25 minutes
Cooking Time: 35 minutes
Servings: 04
Ingredients:

- For the Crust
- Cold water
- Agave, splash
- Sea salt, pinch
- Grapeseed oil, .5 c
- Coconut flour, .5 c
- Spelt Flour, 1 c
- For the Filling
- Butternut squash, peeled, chopped
- Water
- Allspice, to taste
- Agave syrup, to taste
- Hemp milk, 1 c
- Sea moss, 4 tbsp.

Directions:

1. You will need to warm your oven to 350.
2. For the Crust
3. Place the grapeseed oil and water into the refrigerator to get it cold. This will take about one hour.
4. Place all **Ingredients** into a large bowl. Now you need to add in the cold water a little bit in small amounts until a dough forms. Place this onto a surface that has been sprinkled with some coconut flour. Knead for a few minutes and roll the dough as thin as you can get it. Carefully, pick it up and place it inside a pie plate.

5. Place the butternut squash into a Dutch oven and pour in enough water to cover. Bring this to a full rolling boil. Let this cook until the squash has become soft.
6. Completely drain and place into bowl. Using a potato masher, mash the squash. Add in some allspice and agave to taste. Add in the sea moss and hemp milk. Using a hand mixer, blend well. Pour into the pie crust.
7. Place into an oven and bake for about one hour.

Nutrition:

- Calories: 245
- Carbohydrates: 50 g
- Fat: 10 g

88. Coconut Chia Cream Pot

Preparation Time: 5 minutes
Cooking Time: 5 minutes
Servings: 04
Ingredients:

- Date, one (1)
- Coconut milk (organic), one (1) cup
- Coconut yogurt, one (1) cup
- Vanilla extract, ½ teaspoon
- Chia seeds, ¼ cup
- Sesame seeds, one (1) teaspoon
- Flaxseed (ground), one (1) tablespoon or flax meal, one (1) tablespoon
- Toppings:
- Fig, one (1)
- Blueberries, one(1) handful
- Mixed nuts (brazil nuts, almonds, pistachios, macadamia, etc.)
- Cinnamon (ground), one teaspoon

Directions:

1. First, blend the date with coconut milk (the idea is to sweeten the coconut milk).
2. Get a mixing bowl and add the coconut milk with the vanilla, sesame seeds, chia seeds, and flax meal.

3. Refrigerate for between twenty to thirty minutes or wait till the chia expands.
4. To serve, pour a layer of coconut yogurt in a small glass, then add the chia mix, followed by pouring another layer of the coconut yogurt.
5. It's alkaline, creamy and delicious.

Nutrition:

- Calories: 310
- Carbohydrates: 39 g
- Protein: 4 g
- Fiber: 8.1 g

89. Pumpkin & Banana Ice Cream

Preparation Time: 5 minutes
Cooking Time: 10 minutes
Servings: 4
Ingredients:

- 15 oz. pumpkin puree
- 4 bananas, sliced and frozen
- 1 teaspoon pumpkin pie spice
- Chopped pecans

Directions:

1. Add pumpkin puree, bananas and pumpkin pie spice in a food processor.
2. Pulse until smooth.
3. Chill in the refrigerator.
4. Garnish with pecans.

Nutrition:

- 71 Calories
- 18g Carbohydrate; 1.2g Protein

90. Brulee Oranges

Preparation Time: 5 minutes
Cooking Time: 10 minutes
Servings: 4
Ingredients:

- 4 oranges, sliced into segments
- 1 teaspoon ground cardamom
- 6 teaspoons brown sugar
- 1 cup nonfat Greek yogurt

Directions:

1. Preheat your broiler.
2. Arrange orange slices in a baking pan.
3. In a bowl, mix the cardamom and sugar.
4. Sprinkle mixture on top of the oranges. Broil for 5 minutes.
5. Serve oranges with yogurt.

Nutrition:

- 168 Calories
- 26.9g Carbohydrate
- 6.8g Protein

91. Chocolate Crunch Bars

Preparation Time: 5 minutes
Cooking Time: 5 minutes
Servings: 4
Ingredients:

- 1 1/2 cups sugar-free chocolate chips
- 1 cup almond butter
- Stevia to taste
- 1/4 cup coconut oil
- 3 cups pecans, chopped

Directions:

1. Layer an 8-inch baking pan with parchment paper.
2. Mix chocolate chips with butter, coconut oil, and sweetener in a bowl.
3. Melt it by heating in a microwave for 2 to 3 minutes until well mixed.

4. Stir in nuts and seeds. Mix gently.
5. Pour this batter carefully into the baking pan and spread evenly.
6. Refrigerate for 2 to 3 hours.
7. Slice and serve.

Nutrition:

- Calories 316
- Total Fat 30.9 g
- Saturated Fat 8.1 g
- Cholesterol 0 mg
- Total Carbs 8.3 g
- Sugar 1.8 g
- Fiber 3.8 g
- Sodium 8 mg
- Protein 6.4 g

92. Homemade Protein Bar

Preparation Time: 5 minutes
Cooking Time: 10 minutes
Servings: 4
Ingredients:
- 1 cup nut butter
- 4 tablespoons coconut oil
- 2 scoops vanilla protein
- Stevia, to taste
- ½ teaspoon sea salt
- Optional **Ingredients:**
- 1 teaspoon cinnamon

Directions:
1. Mix coconut oil with butter, protein, stevia, and salt in a dish.
2. Stir in cinnamon and chocolate chip.
3. Press the mixture firmly and freeze until firm.
4. Cut the crust into small bars.
5. Serve and enjoy.

Nutrition:

- Calories 179
- Total Fat 15.7 g
- Saturated Fat 8 g
- Cholesterol 0 mg
- Total Carbs 4.8 g
- Sugar 3.6 g
- Fiber 0.8 g
- Sodium 43 mg, Protein 5.6 g

93. Shortbread Cookies

Preparation Time: 10 minutes
Cooking Time: 70 minutes
Servings: 6
Ingredients:

- 2 1/2 cups almond flour
- 6 tablespoons nut butter
- 1/2 cup erythritol
- 1 teaspoon vanilla essence

Directions:

1. Preheat your oven to 350 degrees F.
2. Layer a cookie sheet with parchment paper.
3. Beat butter with erythritol until fluffy.
4. Stir in vanilla essence and almond flour. Mix well until becomes crumbly.
5. Spoon out a tablespoon of cookie dough onto the cookie sheet.
6. Add more dough to make as many cookies.
7. Bake for 15 minutes until brown.
8. Serve.

Nutrition:

- Calories 288
- Total Fat 25.3 g
- Saturated Fat 6.7 g
- Cholesterol 23 mg

- Total Carbs 9.6 g
- Sugar 0.1 g
- Fiber 3.8 g
- Sodium 74 mg
- Potassium 3 mg
- Protein 7.6 g

94. Coconut Chip Cookies

Preparation Time: 10 minutes
Cooking Time: 15 minutes
Servings: 4
Ingredients:
- 1 cup almond flour
- ½ cup cacao nibs
- ½ cup coconut flakes, unsweetened
- 1/3 cup erythritol
- ½ cup almond butter
- ¼ cup nut butter, melted
- ¼ cup almond milk
- Stevia, to taste
- ¼ teaspoon sea salt

Directions:
1. Preheat your oven to 350 degrees F.
2. Layer a cookie sheet with parchment paper.
3. Add and then combine all the dry **Ingredients** in a glass bowl.
4. Whisk in butter, almond milk, vanilla essence, stevia, and almond butter.
5. Beat well then stir in dry mixture. Mix well.
6. Spoon out a tablespoon of cookie dough on the cookie sheet.
7. Add more dough to make as many as 16 cookies.
8. Flatten each cookie using your fingers.
9. Bake for 25 minutes until golden brown.
10. Let them sit for 15 minutes.
11. Serve.

Nutrition:

- Calories 192
- Total Fat 17.44 g
- Saturated Fat 11.5 g
- Cholesterol 125 mg
- Total Carbs 2.2 g
- Sugar 1.4 g
- Fiber 2.1 g
- Sodium 135 mg
- Protein 4.7 g

95. Peanut Butter Bars

Preparation Time: 10 minutes
Cooking Time: 10 minutes
Servings: 6
Ingredients:
- 3/4 cup almond flour
- 2 oz. almond butter
- 1/4 cup Swerve
- 1/2 cup peanut butter
- 1/2 teaspoon vanilla

Directions:
1. Combine all the **Ingredients** for bars.
2. Transfer this mixture to 6-inch small pan. Press it firmly.
3. Refrigerate for 30 minutes.
4. Slice and serve.

Nutrition:

- Calories 214
- Total Fat 19 g
- Saturated Fat 5.8 g
- Cholesterol 15 mg

- Total Carbs 6.5 g
- Sugar 1.9 g
- Fiber 2.1 g
- Sodium 123 mg
- Protein 6.5 g

96. Zucchini Bread Pancakes

Preparation Time: 15 minutes
Cooking Time: 35 minutes
Servings: 3
Ingredients:

- Grapeseed oil, 1 tbsp.
- Chopped walnuts, .5 c
- Walnut milk, 2 c
- Shredded zucchini, 1 c
- Mashed burro banana, .25 c
- Date sugar, 2 tbsp.
- Kamut flour or spelt, 2 c

Directions:
1. Place the date sugar and flour into a bowl. Whisk together.
2. Add in the mashed banana and walnut milk. Stir until combined. Remember to scrape the bowl to get all the dry mixture. Add in walnuts and zucchini. Stir well until combined.
3. Place the grapeseed oil onto a griddle and warm.
4. Pour .25 cup batter on the hot griddle. Leave it along until bubbles begin forming on to surface. Carefully turn over the pancake and cook another four minutes until cooked through.
5. Place the pancakes onto a serving plate and enjoy with some agave syrup.

Nutrition:

- Calories: 246
- Carbohydrates: 49.2 g
- Fiber: 4.6 g
- Protein: 7.8 g

97. Berry Sorbet

Preparation Time: 10 minutes
Cooking Time: 20 minutes
Servings: 6
Ingredients:

- Water, 2 c
- Blend strawberries, 2 c
- Spelt Flour, 1.5 tsp.
- Date sugar, .5 c

Directions:

1. Add the water into a large pot and let the water begin to warm. Add the flour and date sugar and stir until dissolved. Allow this mixture to start boiling and continue to cook for around ten minutes. It should have started to thicken. Take off the heat and set to the side to cool.
2. Once the syrup has cooled off, add in the strawberries, and stir well to combine.
3. Pour into a container that is freezer safe and put it into the freezer until frozen.
4. Take sorbet out of the freezer, cut into chunks, and put it either into a blender or a food processor. Hit the pulse button until the mixture is creamy.
5. Pour this into the same freezer-safe container and put it back into the freezer for four hours.

Nutrition:

- Calories: 99
- Carbohydrates: 8 g

98. Quinoa Porridge

Preparation Time: 5 minutes
Cooking Time: 15 minutes
Servings: 04
Ingredients:

- Zest of one lime

- Coconut milk, .5 c
- Cloves, .5 tsp.
- Ground ginger, 1.5 tsp.
- Spring water, 2 c
- Quinoa, 1 c
- Grated apple, 1

Directions:
1. Cook the quinoa. Follow the instructions on the package. When the quinoa has been cooked, drain well. Place it back into the pot and stir in spices.
2. Add coconut milk and stir well to combine.
3. Grate the apple now and stir well.
4. Divide equally into bowls and add the lime zest on top. Sprinkle with nuts and seeds of choice.

Nutrition:

- Calories: 180
- Fat: 3 g
- Carbohydrates: 40 g
- Protein: 10 g

99. Apple Quinoa

Preparation Time: 15 minutes
Cooking Time: 30 minutes
Servings: 04
Ingredients:
- Coconut oil, 1 tbsp.
- Ginger
- Key lime .5
- Apple, 1
- Quinoa, .5 c
- Optional toppings
- Seeds
- Nuts
- Berries

Directions:

1. Fix the quinoa according to the instructions on the package. When you are getting close to the end of the **Cooking time**, grate in the apple and cook for 30 seconds.
2. Zest the lime into the quinoa and squeeze the juice in. Stir in the coconut oil.
3. Divide evenly into bowls and sprinkle with some ginger.
4. You can add in some berries, nuts, and seeds right before you eat.

Nutrition:

- Calories: 146
- Fiber: 2.3 g
- Fat: 8.3 g

Conclusion

Type 1 diabetes is all about being proactive, and being able to recognize when your blood sugars are getting too high and when they're too low. There are a lot of people with type 1 diabetes who don't know when their blood sugars are too high or too low or in what range they should be. Type II diabetes is the more common form of diabetes. It accounts for about 90 percent of diabetes cases. Type II diabetes usually occur because a person's body has lost the ability to produce insulin.

Type 1 diabetes occurs because the immune system destroys the insulin-producing cells of the pancreas. In the early stages of the disease, you may experience episodes of low blood sugar, called hypoglycemia, that can be dangerous if they occur frequently.

Having Type 1 diabetes will teach you a load of tough lessons. Only about ¼ of diabetics are Type 1. But I'm here to tell you, even though Type 1 is the most common type of diabetes, Type 2 diabetes can be almost as bad.

Being diagnosed with the disease will bring some major changes in your lifestyle. From the time you are diagnosed with it, it would always be a constant battle with food. You need to become a lot more careful with your food choices and the quantity that you ate. Every meal will feel like a major effort. You will be planning every day for the whole week, well in advance. Depending upon the type of food you ate, you have to keep checking your blood sugar levels. You may get used to taking long breaks between meals and staying away from snacks between dinner and breakfast.

Food would be treated as a bomb like it can go off at any time. According to an old saying, "When the body gets too hot, then your body heads straight to the kitchen."

Managing diabetes can be a very, very stressful ordeal. There will be many times that you will mark your glucose levels down on a piece of paper like you are plotting graph lines or something. You will mix your insulin shots up and then stress about whether or not you are giving yourself the right dosage. You will always be over-cautious because it involves a LOT of math and a really fine margin of error. But now, those days are gone!

With the help of technology and books, you can stock your kitchen with the right foods, like meal plans, diabetic friendly dishes, etc. You can get an app that will even do the work for you. You can also people-watch on the internet and find the know-how to cook and eat right; you will always be a few meals away from certain disasters, like a plummeting blood sugar level. Always carry some sugar in your pocket. You won't have to experience the pangs of hunger but if you are unlucky, you will have to ration your food and bring along some simple low-calorie snacks with you.

As you've reached the end of this book, you have gained complete control of your diabetes and this is just the beginning of your journey towards a better, healthier life.

Regardless of the length or seriousness of your diabetes, it can be managed! Take the information presented here and start with it!

Lightning Source UK Ltd.
Milton Keynes UK
UKHW022109110621
385375UK00002B/287